Stealing Second Base

*A Breast Cancer Survivor's Experience
and Breast Cancer Expert's Story*

Lillie Shockney, RN, BS, MAS

Administrative Director
Johns Hopkins Avon Foundation Breast Center
and Johns Hopkins Cancer Survivorship Programs

University Distinguished Service Associate Professor of Breast Cancer

Associate Professor
Johns Hopkins University School of Medicine
Departments of Surgery, Oncology, and Gynecology and Obstetrics

Associate Professor
Johns Hopkins University School of Nursing

Baltimore, MD

JONES AND BARTLETT PUBLISHERS
Sudbury, Massachusetts
BOSTON   TORONTO   LONDON   SINGAPORE

World Headquarters
Jones and Bartlett
Publishers
40 Tall Pine Drive
Sudbury, MA 01776
info@jbpub.com
www.jbpub.com

Jones and Bartlett Publishers
Canada
6339 Ormindale Way
Mississauga, Ontario L5V 1J2
CANADA

Jones and Bartlett Publishers
International
Barb House, Barb Mews
London W6 7PA
UK

Jones and Bartlett's books and products are available through most bookstores and online booksellers. To contact Jones and Bartlett Publishers directly, call 800-832-0034, fax 978-443-8000, or visit our website, www.jbpub.com.

Substantial discounts on bulk quantities of Jones and Bartlett's publications are available to corporations, professional associations, and other qualified organizations. For details and specific discount information, contact the special sales department at Jones and Bartlett via the above contact information or send an email to specialsales@jbpub.com.

The author, editor, and publisher have made every effort to provide accurate information. However, they are not responsible for errors, omissions, or for any outcomes related to the use of the contents of this book and take no responsibility for the use of the products described. Treatments and side effects described in this book may not be applicable to all patients; likewise, some patients may require a dose or experience a side effect that is not described herein. The reader should confer with his or her own physician regarding specific treatments and side effects. Drugs and medical devices are discussed that may have limited availability controlled by the Food and Drug Administration (FDA) for use only in a research study or clinical trial. The drug information presented has been derived from reference sources, recently published data, and pharmaceutical research data. Research, clinical practice, and government regulations often change the accepted standard in this field. When consideration is being given to use of any drug in the clinical setting, the healthcare provider or reader is responsible for determining FDA status of the drug, reading the package insert, reviewing prescribing information for the most up-to-date recommendations on dose, precautions, and contraindications, and determining the appropriate usage for the product. This is especially important in the case of drugs that are new or seldom used.

Copyright © 2007 by Jones and Bartlett Publishers, Inc.

Library of Congress Cataloging-in-Publication Data
Shockney, Lillie, 1953-
    Stealing second base: a breast cancer survivor's experience and breast cancer expert's story / Lillie Shockney.
        p. cm.
    ISBN-13: 978-0-7637-4509-7 (pbk.)
    ISBN-10: 0-7637-4509-X
    1. Shockney, Lillie, 1953- 2. Breast--Cancer--Patients--United States--Biography. 3. Breast--Cancer--Popular works. I. Title.
    RC280.B8S49525 2007
    362.196'994490092—dc22
    [B]
                                    2006017425
6048

Production Credits
Executive Publisher: Christopher Davis
Associate Editor: Kathy Richardson
Production Director: Amy Rose
Associate Production Editor: Kate Hennessy
Production Editor: Carolyn F. Rogers
Associate Marketing Manager: Laura Kavigian
Manufacturing Buyer: Therese Connell
Composition: Northeast Compositors, Inc.
Cover Design: Kristin E. Ohlin
Cover Image: © Ambidox/ShutterStock, Inc.
Interior Images: © Image Club Graphics
Senior Photo Researcher: Kimberly Potvin
Printing and Binding: Malloy, Inc.
Cover Printing: Malloy, Inc.

Printed in the United States of America
16 15 14 13 12   10 9 8 7 6 5

This book is dedicated to

—my husband, Al, for demonstrating his undying love for me
—my daughter, Laura, who has grown into an amazing young woman as well as
   my best friend
—my parents for teaching me that anything is possible if you work hard enough
—future breast cancer survivors who may end up wearing my bra

Contents

Introduction

The decision about the title of this book was made long before any thoughts were put to paper. And though it may not sound like a book related to breast cancer and breast reconstruction, "second base" has had meaning to my generation and several generations before me. So for those of you in my generation (I was born in 1953), you may remember as a teen listening inquisitively on Monday morning to high school girls discussing their weekend dates. "How far did you let him get? Did he get to second base?"—the famous breast zone. I always found it fascinating that the body was divided up like a baseball field. We were of course taught to stay away from the boys who were hell bent on hitting home runs and that only girls who were respected didn't let boys get to any bases at all. I never participated in the discussions but found it amazing the importance girls placed in reporting "the scores" on Monday mornings to their giggly friends.

"Did he get to second base?"—the famous breast zone.

We are taught when we are young the importance of breasts. Society molds us early on. I have a photograph of a child, about 10, standing on the beach with a woman about 30. They are both wearing t-shirts and have their heads tilted back, drinking in the sunshine, their chests proudly protruding, as if making their own statement without words. But there ARE words on the child's t-shirt. It says "Watch This Space." And we do…The woman's t-shirt says nothing. It doesn't need to—her large breasts speak volumes without having to make written billboards on her clothing.

I had every intention of making sure my own daughter, Laura, didn't get molded by society when it came to breasts and women's bodies, and I learned when she was just 3 years of age that I had failed at this attempt before she even started kindergarten. For several consecutive nights she had awakened during the night crying, saying that her chest hurt, and pointing to her nipples. I inspected them closely, finding them red and hot. When I touched them, she winced. After I would sit with her on her bed for a few minutes, talk with her, and sing to her, she would go back to sleep. In the morning the redness and heat were gone. But for 6 nights this pattern continued until I officially diagnosed her with pediatric nocturnal mastitis. (Yes, I am a nurse.) So off to the pediatrician we went, weary of not getting sleep and anxious to have my diagnosis confirmed and of course treated. The doctor was not surprised I had determined what my child had, but promptly burst my bubble by telling me there was no such thing. After he examined her, he proceeded to ask Laura questions I had failed to ask her myself. "Laura, have you been pulling on your nipples after you go to bed at night?" She responded, nodding her head affirmatively. I was stunned. He continued, "Tell me why you have been doing this." Laura said, "Because I want my boobies to grow big like mommy's." Now I'm in shock. Boobies? Where had she heard such a word? The pediatrician proceeded to calmly and without surprise say, "Well, pulling on them makes them sore and that's why they hurt and you have trouble sleeping. If you eat lots of green vegetables, they will grow to be even bigger than your mommy's." To this day my child, now age 26, has no clue why she has loved broccoli and green beans since a toddler. And yes, whether scientific, genetic, or just coincidence, her breasts are large, just like mine used to be ... which takes me to my story.

CHAPTER ONE

You Have Breast Cancer

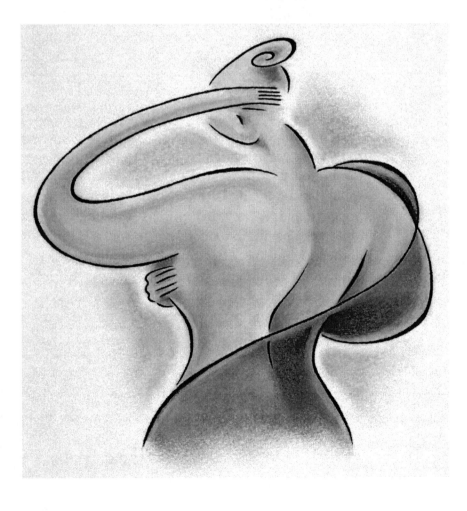

Most women hear these words from their doctor, who is trying to gently break the news that they have just been diagnosed. My situation was different. I was overly confident that my biopsy would be benign, so I pulled up my own pathology report while my surgeon was out of town. I read "breast carcinoma" 12 times. I couldn't believe it was my report, my name, my history number, and I badly wanted it to belong to anyone else. But it wasn't someone else's; it was mine and I had to take ownership of it. I have no recall of driving home that evening but do remember walking out of the hospital. I routinely used the main entrance of the hospital to go in and out. The lobby area is a national landmark. This is where the statue of Christ is standing with arms stretched out. I, as many passersby do, always touched His right great toe as I entered and exited. Not that night, however. I was hesitant to even look up at His face and moved by the statue swiftly, afraid He might turn and speak to me before I was ready for a discussion about my mortality that I now was in touch with in a frightening way. He and I would need to talk later when I could collect my thoughts and know what prayers I wanted to say. Some people say, "Be careful what you ask for." My mother taught me, "Be careful what you pray for." Wise words. I certainly wasn't going to ask Christ to take the cancer away. I did, however, want to ask for strength to endure whatever lay ahead for me and for my family.

Driving home from work that evening remains a part of my past that is erased. I have no idea how I managed to do it and hope that I didn't scare anyone in my path. I knew my husband would not be home for several more hours and that he had no idea I had planned to access my pathology report. So I thought I should practice how I would tell him that his wife in fact had breast cancer. I stood in front of the bathroom mirror and rehearsed what I would say. Explaining that I had access to the pathology database, that mom was calling me every day asking me if I knew anything yet, that I felt sure I would read benign results, but didn't, and that I did have breast cancer. While standing in the bathroom, I imagined hundreds of people walking through my house on the day of my burial and silently commenting how messy the bathroom was. So, I did what probably many women in a state of panic and delusion would do. I proceeded to clean my house head to toe and help the time pass until my husband got home. When I finished, I looked around and now imagined people saying, "Well, from diagnosis to death was only a week. Wow. But didn't she keep a nice clean house" (as if that was important right now).

When the kitchen door opened at 11:30 that night and my husband walked through it, rather than reciting to him the words I had rehearsed in the mirror so many times that night, I instead burst out "I have breast cancer." He was stunned, confused, and asked if my surgeon had returned from his trip. I then explained what I had done and how I knew my situation. He put his arms around me and asked if I knew how bad it was. I told him that I didn't, yet I should. I translate pathology reports for people, but seeing this report with my name and history number on it and words that were so terribly frightening to me, I elected to not even print it out and hoped it evaporated in the computer system during the night. Perhaps when I went to work in the morning, a new report would appear saying, "Ha ha, fooled you. That will teach you to look up your own report." But I knew that wasn't the case. … I had flipped to the other side of the side rail, going from a nurse to a cancer patient in a matter of seconds. He reassured me and told me that whatever lay ahead we would beat it together, and I held onto those words.

When my surgeon returned 3 days later, I told him that I knew what my pathology report said but wasn't sure what the treatment requirements were going to be, though subconsciously I knew all along. Mastectomy.

I was diagnosed with this particular breast cancer at the age of 38. As is the case for most women, I had no known risk factors, but 70% of women diagnosed today fit that description. Mine was found coincidentally. I had a lump in my right breast, prompting me to get a mammogram. That lump was a cyst, but a baseline mammogram was taken of my left breast since I was between the ages of 35 and 40, and there they found what would alter the rest of my life in more ways than imaginable. After a wire localization open surgical biopsy was performed, I learned I had stage 1 breast cancer, but extensive ductal carcinoma in situ accompanied these findings. Despite having large breasts (my bra size was 44D), I was advised to have a mastectomy due to multicentric disease—having more than one area in my breast with cancer in it. I was also advised not to pursue reconstruction at the time because of a history of serious anesthesia complications (respiratory arrests). Keep it simple was the message.

Simple wasn't easy though. Part of my self-image was tied up on my chest. I was identified in a crowd based on my breast size—"Go over to the woman with the large breasts; she will assist you." I worried about how I would look at my new self-image and worried even more what impact it would have on my sexuality and my marriage. Once I came to grips with the concept of the disease itself and that I would survive it, I did as many women do—looked at the ripple effect this would have on my life and how I perceived that impact.

As a nurse I had taken care of many women with breast cancer during my nursing career. I understood it was the most feared disease of all women, and I shared that fear, though I never imagined becoming diagnosed with it myself. Suddenly I felt like I was a man in a woman's body, looking at other women's breasts while grocery shopping, buying shoes, or picking my child up after school. I wondered if I could spot other women who had had mastectomies like I was soon to have. Do they evenly bounce the same way? Are they symmetric and the same size? Can the nipples be seen? Those were all distinctive features I thought would be able to tell me the secret of how to find another mastectomy patient without her wearing a sign saying she had had such surgery. Cleavage had new meaning because I was about to see mine leave town and not return. But, despite this, my focus was primarily on survival ... being there for my daughter and my family. If the surgeon had told me that I needed to lose my arm with my breast, I would have agreed if it would guarantee me longevity. When we hear the words "you have breast cancer," foxhole religion usually takes hold. You hear those bullets sailing overhead and will do whatever it takes to get to safe ground. I thought I knew a lot about breast cancer and its treatment, but being on the other side of the side rail provided me with a perspective that is hard to explain. I had found a new way of thinking about the patients I had taken care of in the past, and I also knew that my career path would soon change as a result too, steering me back in the direction of taking care of women who ended up wearing my bra after me. (I used to say I took care of women who walked in my footsteps, but I haven't had foot surgery so I don't say that anymore.)

At the time I was diagnosed, considerable time had passed since I had taken care of women with this disease. My nursing career had led me down a different professional track for the last few years, away from bedside care. I didn't feel in touch with what to expect, what I would look like, and how I would feel. I rapidly began to refresh my memory and get updated on the newest treatments, what the surgical procedure would entail, and what additional concerns I may need to face, such as recurrence, adjuvant therapy, and coping in general. My strongest memories were of women I had taken care of in the recovery room as a student nurse, memories I will never forget that haunt me to this day. This was at a time that we had women sign an operative consent form to have a breast biopsy done under general anesthesia and have the specimen sent for frozen section to pathology. If found to be cancer, they awakened in the recovery room, having had a total radical mastectomy—breast and chest muscles gone. I remember the first patient I took care of who had had such a procedure done. She awakened and said to me, "Please, please tell me my breast isn't gone. Please tell me he didn't take it off." And I froze because it was gone. I was just 17 years old. My silence expressed her worst fear, and she began to sob. I cried too, not having any idea how to help or console this patient. I remember calling my mother that night and telling her about it. She responded by telling me that she predicted at some point in my nursing career I would have an opportunity to improve the surgical experience for women undergoing breast cancer surgery. Little did I know she was predicting my future and that I too would become a patient in order to effect such improvements for others coming behind me. Isn't it good we really don't have a crystal ball to see our future in detail? It would be emotionally impossible to cope with.

CHAPTER TWO

So What's So Funny about Getting Breast Cancer?

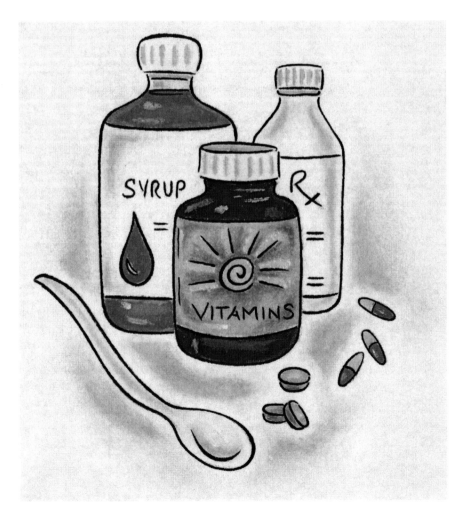

Laura, our daughter, was 12 when I was diagnosed. I had just had her fitted for her first bra the same week as my breast biopsy, so breasts were on her mind once again. I waited several days before breaking the news to her, wanting to see my surgeon and having a plan before discussing it with her. She asked two questions of me. Because patients had been kind enough to share with me their own children's questions, I was prepared with answers. She asked, "Mommy, are you going to die?" I told her that I had stage 1 breast cancer and had an excellent prognosis and that after all she would soon become a teenager and did she believe God would leave daddy here alone to raise her by himself? She said, "No, God wouldn't do that to daddy. I've already made his hair turn white and I think that would make it fall out." I agreed. Then she asked me a question that children between the ages of 4 and 13 often think about but are hesitant to verbalize. She said, "Did you get breast cancer because you had me?" I explained to her that having her when I was 26 helped reduce my risk of getting breast cancer because if you have your first child when you are under the age of 30 it helps to reduce the risk of getting this disease. That relieved her.

Then she asked me questions I had no anticipated answer for. Here they are: "Will the doctor let you bring your breast home to keep? After all it isn't his, it's yours. You could put it in daddy's big pickle jar and keep it on the mantle and when you are sad you could go and look at it." I asked Al, "What do you think, honey? My breast in a pickle jar next to your deer head and blue fish?" He said, "We'd have to get a bigger pickle jar because I don't have one big enough to hold your breast." Then she asked me, "Will the doctor move your right breast to the middle?" Wow. Take a look at the operative consent form carefully for this surgical treatment. I told her I didn't plan on him rearranging the other one and asked her why she thought that might be part of the surgical treatment. She said, "Well, if he doesn't, you are going to lean to the right when you walk." I explained to her that I would be wearing a breast prosthesis inside of a mastectomy bra that had a pocket in it and showed her a photograph in a mastectomy supply catalog of what this looked like. She said, "A bra with a pocket. What a clever thing. You always worry when you go to the ATM bank machine that someone will steal your money. You could put it in that pocket, then no one can get it." My husband said, "Excellent suggestion. I hate waiting in those long lines with you at the grocery store. You can start getting your money out, and we can make an express line wherever we want to."

What Laura had done for us was find our sense of humor. Her questions were serious to her but hit our funny bone in the perfect way, and we made a pact that every day for the rest of our lives we would find something funny about the fact I had been diagnosed. And trust me, we do.

Until I told our daughter about my situation, there was no laughter in our house. Five days had passed since I had learned I had breast cancer. It was 3 days after reading my pathology report before my surgeon was back in town to discuss what needed to be done to get me well again. What was strange was I didn't feel sick, again typical of this disease. Laura's wonderful questions brought a new perspective to the situation. It helped me reflect back on my own childhood at her age. Ironically at the same age, 12, I had my first experience with breast cancer. That's when my mother's best friend, Miss Bertha, was diagnosed with this disease. Though a well-educated woman, a psychologist, she didn't know the warning signs of a breast health problem. She had an open draining sore on her breast and a mass the size of a softball for more than a year before she sought medical care. She only went to the doctor then because her ribs were sore. "My ribs really bother me. I must be getting arthritis at an early age." She was 55. She decided to see her doctor to get some "arthritis ointment." Needless to say that is not what he prescribed. He examined her, did a series of tests, and explained to her that she had advanced metastatic breast cancer. Her ribs hurt because it had spread to her ribs, and to her hip joint, her lungs, and her liver. The tumor had actually grown so large it had broken through the skin.

Her doctor told her he would treat her aggressively, performing a total radical mastectomy (a procedure developed by Dr. William Halsted a century ago at Johns Hopkins). He would follow this with chemotherapy (we had only one drug to offer then) and radiation to her entire body. But he was frank in saying that he didn't expect her to survive to see treatment completed. He estimated she would live approximately 5 months, urging her to go home and get her affairs in order. She told him that she didn't have time to get her affairs in order because she was going to be too busy living. She explained that she had made a list of the personal goals she intended to achieve before she left this world and she had just decided to add an additional goal to the list—that goal was to outlive him, her doctor! And Miss Bertha did. She survived for 21 more years. (By the way, her doctor died of a heart attack 18 years after her diagnosis, so she accomplished her goal.)

She was amazing and a wonderful mentor for me at a time when I had no clue how significant her attitude about this disease would have on my future and my own personal health. A key lesson she taught me was the value of humor. She said, "I think that humor builds the immune system, and it is the immune system that has gone on the blink to allow cancer cells to grow. So I'm going to find something to laugh about every day as part of my treatment." She was 35 years ahead of research later done to prove her hypothesis was right.

She did everything her doctors told her to do except for one thing—she didn't do her arm exercises: walking up the walls with your fingers, swinging a dowel stick over your head—all a waste of time in her mind. When she was 7 weeks post-op and couldn't raise her arm up over her head, she realized maybe those exercises had a purpose after all. But they were boring and to be done indoors. She told me, "I know I need to get my range of motion and arm strength back, so I'm going to take up golf where I can enjoy the fresh air and hear the birds sing." She hired a young man named David, just 25 years old, as her instructor. David actually thought she was interested in the sport, but she was not. Every Wednesday she would have a class with him, and every Saturday I would get to see her. She would basically tell me the same thing each weekend. "David yelled at me again. He says I'm not swinging my arm all the way through." I told her, "Miss Bertha, why don't you simply tell him that

"I think that humor builds the immune system, and it is the immune system that has gone on the blink to allow cancer cells to grow. So I'm going to find something to laugh about every day as part of my treatment." She was 35 years ahead of research later done to prove her hypothesis was right.

13

you've had an operation." She was horrified at the thought of having this be known. This was 40 years ago when breast cancer was a hushed disease. We didn't discuss it in public and frankly barely discussed it in private. So she declined to tell him her troubles.

Eight weeks into her lessons when I saw her that Saturday, she acted very differently. "I did it! I did it! I finally did it! I decided this past Wednesday that David wasn't going to yell at me. I connected with the ball, both of my arms went all the way up, and I couldn't believe how far that ball had gone and that I was the one to whack it so far! Then I looked down and saw my breast prosthesis at my feet." Yes, this was before we had mastectomy bras with pockets in them to hold a prosthesis securely in place. Miss Bertha's arms went up and this object flipped out from the front neck opening of her shirt, landing squarely between them. She said, "We both just stared at it. I didn't want to pick it up and claim it. I wanted to tell David it belonged to the people playing golf up ahead of us, but there were no people up ahead of us. Then David reached down, picked it up, and said to me, 'Why didn't you tell me you have had surgery. Is this why you are having trouble with your arm?' He made me feel comfortable at a time I otherwise would have felt very embarrassed." I was so proud of this young man who I never met and haven't ever seen to this day. He took the vulnerability away from her. He made her feel it was okay to be one-breasted. He also turned her into a wonderful golf player. Within 3 years Miss Bertha had trophies lined up on her mantel, and I felt that each of them was courtesy of David.

Miss Bertha had a friend named Lena. She lived in Rochester, originally where Miss Bertha was from. I was accustomed to seeing Lena in the month of July when she would come down to stay for a week, vacationing with Miss Bertha at her home. I noticed, though, after Miss Bertha's surgery, Lena was coming down every other weekend, driving down on a Friday and returning home on Monday. Then during a weekend when I was visiting Miss Bertha I realized why. Lena was also a breast cancer survivor. She had been diagnosed with breast cancer 2 years before Miss Bertha and had had bilateral mastectomies. She was spending time with her to offer her support. This was long before there were support groups and decades before breast cancer was discussed in public. It remained a private nightmare for women. It was comforting to know that Miss Bertha had a comrade to talk with regarding personal concerns she had related to this disease and its treatment. When Lena heard what had happened to Miss Bertha out on the golf course, she said, "Oh, Bertha. I feel responsible for that. I should have told you, if you aren't careful, these things will get away." And Lena was certainly one who would know because she was a gymnastics teacher. But not your typical gymnast. Lena was 6 feet tall and very large busted. I had the opportunity to see her do a gymnastics routine one time and was very impressed with how agile she was on her feet. She said, "The first time I returned to work, I was in the gym with a class of 5th grade girls, showing them how to do cartwheels. I got into the third cartwheel and both of my prostheses skid across the floor, flying right out of my bra and shirt. It scared the girls to death. I realized then that I wouldn't be able to wear my prostheses to work. I didn't want to just rely on my husband's socks in my bra though because they had no weight. So I decided to drive into New York City, where I found a very unique store that carried inflatable bras." I heard this story at the age of 12 and thought, wow, what a unique store! I'm now 52 and have come to realize that every city has at least one of these stores and they have other inflatable things in them too. There was Lena with her inflated bra on and, trust me, you would never have guessed that she just had air on her chest. She looked quite lovely.

On a weekend that she was visiting and I also had the good fortune to be there with Miss Bertha, she had an interesting story she shared with us. She said, "Well, since I was last here with you, I've had a very unique experience with my inflatable bra. I got on an airplane with it. I saw all the usual signs—no smoking, wear your seat belt. Here's the flotation device in case the plane crashes. But nowhere was there a sign that said, 'if you are wearing an inflatable bra, we strongly rec-ommend you deflate it before takeoff because if you don't when we reach 25,000 feet the sucker is going to explode.'" Yes, you guessed it. She said that the plane started climbing and she was talking to the man sitting next to her, telling him she was traveling from Rochester to Chicago to help her brother move from an apartment into a house, when her chest started vibrating. She said that she looked at her vibrating chest and the man looked at her quivering chest. She attempted to continue the conversation, not even knowing what she was saying, but it didn't matter because he was in shock. Sure enough, before she could get herself back to the bathroom, both breasts blew like a pair of bombs. She scurried back to the lavatory and tried to get her clothes off in that little tiny space. She said she got off her sweater, then her turtleneck, then her exploded bra and checked the damage. Major blowouts right through the nipples.

She then sat on the toilet seat, got out her sewing kit from her purse, stuffed Kleenex in through the nipple holes and sewed the nipple area shut, reassembled herself, and decided to return to her seat and make believe nothing had happened. She attempted to pick up the conversation where she had left off. But apparently while she had been in the bathroom, the man sitting next to her had lost all peripheral vision and gone deaf. He wasn't going to look at her or listen to her! She chalked it up as a day in the life of a breast cancer survivor. I never get on an airplane without thinking about Lena! How wonderful that she could find humor in such an embarrassing moment.

I had the opportunity, really the gift, of getting to speak to Miss Bertha about 2 hours before she passed away. Her sister was taking care of her and called me at Miss Bertha's request. It was difficult to say goodbye but also a moment of reflection for us both, realizing the remarkable journey she had taken ... and how fortunate I was to have been allowed to walk alongside of her for parts of that journey. She told me that she was thankful to have had me in her life and that she was especially grateful that I had been her "borrowed daughter" and not her biological daughter. (She did not have children but badly wanted them. I filled that need in her life.) When I asked her why she was glad I was borrowed and not hers by blood, she said, "I wouldn't have wanted to have worried, thinking I could have passed this disease genetically onto you." Little did either of us know that I had breast cancer then but simply hadn't been diagnosed yet.

CHAPTER THREE

Preparing for the Big Day— Transformation Day

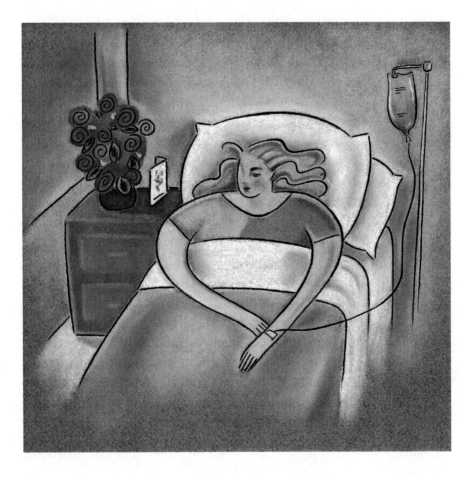

My surgery was scheduled for 8 weeks after I got the news that mastectomy surgery would become part of my medical history. I was not like most women newly diagnosed, anxious for surgery to happen tomorrow and visiting bookstores to see if there was a "do-it-yourself" guide to self-mastectomy if the surgery isn't scheduled quickly. I knew it was safe to wait and knew that this cancer had been there several years. Yes, usually breast cancer has been present quite a while—5 to 7 years—before being discovered, and even then it is still usually an early diagnosis. Until the body figures out this is something that can do us harm, it doesn't create any signals on a mammogram to be found. That doesn't mean we should get mammograms every 5 years instead of annually though. A subtle difference found by the eye of a radiologist who specializes in breast imaging can save our lives and oftentimes save our breasts too. I chose to delay for two reasons—to get a ton of work done so I wouldn't be fretting every day about work while away and to hold onto my breast for as long as possible, though I felt one had betrayed me. I found it difficult to imagine what I was going to feel like being one-breasted, especially having walked around with 44Ds for a long time. I was known as having "bodacious tah tahs" and soon would just have one "tah."

My husband, Al, was amazingly supportive from the moment I gave him the overwhelming news. He remained focused and steadfast, truly a model husband, and I know many women wish they had the same level of support from their significant sweetie. His focus was on my survival. Whether I had two breasts or one or none meant nothing to him. Having me with him was all he cared about. (It wasn't until some time later that I learned how shaken he was by all this and that he had confided in his older brother, Jack, when times were rough. Jack had lost his wife to cancer a few years before I was diagnosed.) Al persuaded me to look at my mastectomy surgery in a different way. He referred to it as "transformation surgery." He said, "Women look at mastectomy as an amputation of an important part of their body. Granted, women ARE losing something special and dear to them. But I think it is better to look at it as transformation surgery. The surgeon's mission is to transform you from a breast cancer victim into a breast cancer survivor. So you are in essence exchanging your breast for another chance at life and that is surely a fair trade." Wise words. Philosophical words. Not said by a philosopher or health care professional but by a tractor trailer driver who I loved a great deal.

The surgeon's mission is to transform you from a breast cancer victim into a breast cancer survivor.

I worried still about what impact all this would have on us, including our sex life. So I asked him to "make a trade with me"—an expression he knows well and that the outcome is that he will get the short end of the stick. When he asked what I wanted, I told him that I wanted to choose the moment when he saw me with just one breast, and I didn't know when that moment would be but I planned to wait a while. When that moment came, I wanted to see him without his teeth. He has upper dentures, and for our 14 years of marriage I had never seen them out of his head. He looked at me with horror at such a request and asked me how important this was to me. I told him it was terribly important. He closed his eyes and shook my hand, agreeing to fulfill my request though he said that he felt he was going to feel more vulnerable than me. I told him that I anticipated we would feel equally vulnerable to one another and that was my wish. I slept better knowing too that I would get to control that moment.

I saw my surgeon the day before my surgery to ask him a list of questions, taking 90 minutes. He patiently went through each one and at the end asked me just one question. "Lillie, you know you and your husband are going to be just fine. I don't think you are going to have any trouble with your self-image. Do you?" I told him my plan to "wait a while" before letting Al see me with just one breast. He then asked me to "define a while." I told him, "2 months." I didn't tell him what the deal was with Al—what the trade arrangement had been. I felt there was no need to provide that detail. He went, "hhmm," and said nothing else. If your surgeon ever goes "hhmm," beware of what he might be planning for you in your near future (more on that later).

Telling my parents that I, their daughter, had breast cancer may have been one of the most difficult moments of my life. I am close to my folks. My mother is known for being a rock during a crisis. She is truly amazing. But this was more than she could cope with. The only saving grace for me was that I didn't have to make eye contact because I told her over the phone. My father told me later that she sobbed for hours, and frankly I believe he probably did too but men don't talk about such things. Waiting the 8 weeks probably was mentally not helpful to anyone, and if I had to do it again I would have said that work comes second, my health comes first. But that wasn't how I was raised. Work was always first. I was well acquainted with hard work, commitment, and responsibilities, having worked on my parents' farm milking cows and in the fields since age 6. Take care of your obligations before you take care of yourself. I was reared on that motto, and my parents were reared on it too.

I also had to make a decision if I was going to go public with my diagnosis. Al and I discussed this, and we decided it was the right thing to do. Not only would it benefit me in getting support from friends and colleagues, but it would also raise awareness so that perhaps more women would be inspired to get mammograms and see their doctor for clinical breast examinations and check themselves monthly. An interesting phenomenon happens, however, when you do tell others. They can't help it and mean no harm by it, but they stare right at your chest. Perhaps they are curious to see if they can tell which one is causing the trouble or maybe trying to picture what you would look like after surgery. There were times I was tempted to stick a post-it on my left breast area that said, "Stop guessing. It's me."

In preparation for surgery I also spent time with anesthesiology faculty to make decisions about what drugs to use that wouldn't cause me to become critically unstable postoperatively. I sure didn't want to die trying to be saved from a diagnosis of cancer from drug reactions like I had experienced before—compromising my respiratory system and heart. They planned on light sedation rather than snowing me. The preparation and several hours of discussion caused me to envy women who did have an option for reconstruction at the same time. So I brought the issue up with Al and told him that I was wondering if we should explore further the option of reconstruction. He was not keen on doing anything that increased my risk. So I tried to joke with him by saying, "Well, let's look at it this way. If I did a TRAM flap and died on the table, you could lay me out topless in the casket. I could really make a statement! After all, I want everyone to see what I died FOR. Maybe the plastic surgeon could quickly do the nipple reconstruction at the funeral home and tattoo the areola too. That way I'd look finished, right? What do you think?" He looked sternly at me and was not amused. End of conversation. Frankly, I wasn't keen on the TRAM flap anyway. The thought of sacrificing my abdominal muscles had no real appeal, and implants were not something that seems logical to me either, especially given my bra cup size.

The evening before my surgery the house was very quiet. Al had taken Laura to his mom's to spend the night. We watched television for a little while—a distraction really. My anesthesiologist called me and talked a while and asked me to "get a good night's sleep" for him. I told him I would try. We watched a show—probably Prime Time Live or a similar program. They were interviewing a baseball player and his wife. This was a man destined to be as famous as our own Baltimore Orioles Cal Ripken, Jr. He was a pitcher and developed bone cancer in, of all places, his pitching arm. He had surgery, chemotherapy, and radiation, and it was a miracle he got to return to the sport. But on national television when he threw a pitch, he fell to the ground, his arm pathologically fractured. His disease was back with a vengeance. He had to have a four quarter amputation of his arm and shoulder, all the way up to his neck, and more chemo and radiation. There would be no returning to his career now. The reporter said, "You must feel devastated that you can't play baseball anymore. How sad for you." He replied, "No, not sad at all. It wasn't my destiny. It was merely a stepping stone on my journey to my true destiny. Now I travel around the country visiting hospitals where there are young boys who have cancer and hope to get well to become a baseball player. That was my true career I was meant to be doing now." The reporter turned to his wife and said, "He must be dependent on you for everything. To get dressed, cut up his food." His wife interrupted the reporter and said, "He is only dependent on me for my love." My husband looked at this couple in awe and said, "Soon that will be us."

I badly wanted to sleep, as the anesthesiologist requested, but couldn't stop thinking about what I would look like and feel like 24 hours from then. I would put my hand up to my left breast and then pull it back down, not wanting to linger there, yet also wishing there was a way to say goodbye to it that would be appropriate. When we got up at 4:30 the next morning, the house was quiet. I asked Al if we should say a prayer over my breast, take a photo of it, or do something to bid it goodbye. He just put his arms around me and said, "Don't worry, we don't need to do anything right now. Today will be a positive day for both of us."

While driving to the hospital, I was thinking negative thoughts. I finally expressed them out loud. "This is an ungodly hour to have to get up and come to the hospital to have my breast amputated." Al replied, "Babe, we agreed that we would only think positive thoughts today. Today is a good day. You are ridding your body of the source of this disease. Please don't think negatively about it. I'm not. I want you well and home with me again." So I sat there silently thinking these negative thoughts. When we arrived at the hospital, it was 5:30 a.m. He dropped me at the entrance and said he would be inside in just a few minutes, once the car was parked. As I entered the hospital, I was still thinking what an ungodly hour this was for such an awful procedure, and coming down the hallway toward me was Clyde Shallenberger, the hospital chaplain. He came over to me and asked what I was doing here so early and why I didn't look like I was dressed for work. I asked him to tell me first why he was here so early. He explained that he had gotten a call at 2:00 a.m. to come in and be with a family who had to make a decision for their loved one who was in the SICU. They had to make the decision within the hour and he helped them with that decision. He was going to go home and get some more sleep but decided to detour through Labor and Delivery and had perfect timing, getting to see a brand new life brought into this world, and it energized him in such a way that he said he was truly high on life and didn't need any more sleep. Then he asked me why I was here so early, and I told him about my diagnosis and surgery. He said, "I'm getting ready to meet with my boss, the Big G. We will have a discussion about you and I will come and find you later in the recovery room." With that said, my husband arrived and I introduced them. I told Al, "You were right and I was wrong. It is not an ungodly hour. It probably is the perfect hour for this."

Upstairs in the pre-op waiting area were clusters of families waiting for their loved one to leave them and go into surgery. A nurse came out and called my name. I went into the back with her. She read the paperwork about my surgery and glanced at my chest and was speechless for a moment, then went about getting my vital signs and asking the usual questions. I got undressed to put on my hospital gown and, while doing so, one of the anesthesiologists, Laurel Moore, came in to see me. Just as she entered the room, I was removing my bra. I looked up at her and said, "I will never be able to wear this bra again. Wow." She gave me a hug and smiled gently at me. I got to see my husband briefly before going to the operating room. When the surgeon came in to escort me back, my husband gave me a kiss, told me he loved me, and said, "Bring her back to me after you have finished her transformation surgery." As I entered the operating room, I felt frightened and vulnerable. Laurel helped me up onto the table. The room was very cold. Several nurses came over and introduced themselves to me, soft spoken. They were caring, compassionate, and no doubt thankful that they were not in my shoes at that moment. The IV went in. The rest of the anesthesia team came in and the attending anesthesiologist who had spent so much time with me before this day reassured me that all was fine and would go well and for me to think happy thoughts as I went off to sleep. He held my hand. I felt lightheaded and could hear my mother's voice singing a religious song called "He Gazed Up and Smiled on Me." I felt peaceful hearing her voice singing, though I knew she wasn't actually in the room with me. Then the color of the walls turned white, a buzzing noise was in my ears, and I was out. There is no way to measure time when you are under anesthesia. It just passes.

When I awakened in the recovery room, I was unaware at first where I was but very aware that I had had surgery. My chest felt tight. (Back in 1992 we used tight binders to compress the chest, thinking it would help in preventing bleeding and fluid formation. We now know that such constriction isn't necessary.) I could hear a woman to my left crying, and I wanted to try to get off the gurney and go to her, an instinct people who seem born to help others simply cannot control. A nurse came over to me and assured me that the other patient was being taken care of and for me to rest. A few minutes later, as I was awakening more, my chest felt tighter. I motioned for the nurse again and apparently told her that I thought an elephant was standing on my chest. I then told her to "not worry" because it was Dumbo and he was fine. Go figure ... the power of the drugs still working, making me say things that normally would never have been thought. I guess I was Dumbo's mother.

Al was brought into the recovery room a few minutes later. He looked as excited as he did the night our child was born. Beaming. He said, "Oh baby, the transformation surgery was successful. I love you so much." Now in retrospect we realize that no one else knew what we were talking about, and I've always wondered if other patients and their family members thought I had had a sex change.

I was transported up to my inpatient room and en route felt like I was out on a small boat in a big ocean with high winds blowing. You guessed it—I was seasick. Nausea hit me big time, and before I made it to the room I was throwing up. This would be the beginning of a long siege of vomiting that I simply couldn't quite get under control. Any motion or movement activated it, like pushing the "on" button of my stomach. (Today we give patients antiemetics during the surgery to prevent this, thank heavens.)

When I got into my room, my parents were there waiting for me. Mom looked whipped, and dad looked nervous. I think if I had been able to look at her knees I would have noted that they looked worn out—from spending so many hours praying on them. She had contacted many of the churches where she regularly sang solos and requested that I be placed on their prayer lists. I now was hoping that these kind people all over the Eastern Shore of Maryland had added my mother to their prayer lists too.

Al was holding a piece of paper in his hand and said, "I've been given specific instructions to read this poem to you when you got into your hospital room. It is from Laura." The poem read:

Appearance
Nobody's perfect
Just look at me
But if you really think about it
Who wants to be?

Beauty and glamour
Are nice to get
But it's what's inside that counts
You must never forget

I hope you understand
What I've been trying to say
I hope you get well soon
And I love you more each day.
Love,
Laura

Beauty and glamour are nice to get But it's what's inside that counts You must never forget

Hearing these wise words of a 12-year-old was not only comforting but gave me a sense of pride. We had raised her right. She was focusing on what was important. A relief to a mother to know that you have done a good job in parenting.

My evening shift nurse was named Myckie. I had never met her before nor seen her since but will remember her for the rest of my life. The evening was busy. A nurse had called in sick with no one to replace her. Two very ill patients were down the hall, having had Whipple surgery—very complicated surgery for pancreatic cancer, which requires a great deal of nursing care and monitoring. I wanted to be as little bother to Myckie as I possibly could. I felt I was perfectly capable, with my husband's assistance, to measure my intake and output. Of course, there was more output than intake. I declined pain medications, knowing it would only aggravate my nausea more. Myckie came about every hour, checking my measurements, emptying my two Hemovac drains, changing my IV bag. Each time she asked me how I was, and each time like it was rehearsed I said that I "was fine." This continued through the evening shift. I had probably more company than was logical to have, a pitfall when you have surgery in the place where you work and coworkers are worried about you. With each visitor I felt the need to look like all was well, and I didn't feel that way at all. Sort of like being on stage. They all meant well, that I knew. I didn't want to upset anyone. At 10 p.m. my husband needed to head home. He looked as exhausted as I felt. He kissed me goodbye and told me he would return to me at 9 a.m. to take me home. That was the plan. My surgeon was to come by at 6:15 a.m. to do a dressing change before going off to surgery, and Al would arrive a few hours later.

The room was suddenly quiet, and for the first time since my surgery I was alone. Alone to reflect on what had happened to me that day. I was now a breast cancer patient officially with a battle scar across my chest to prove it. I didn't know the status of my lymph nodes yet (today we do sentinel node biopsies and know immediately if cancer is there and can forgo an axillary node dissection the majority of the time—a blessing). I also didn't know how much disease was in the breast. All I knew was that it was gone. I looked down at my feet, and for the first time since I was a young teen I could see my toes. A startling and overwhelming feeling. Myckie returned once again to check my IV and empty my Hemovac drains. It was 10:50 p.m.—time for change of shift. Again Myckie asked me how I was, and I again responded as I had all evening, saying I was fine. She paused a moment and put my side rail down and sat on the side of the bed and looked at me. You know the power of getting eye contact with someone? In the split second when your eyes meet someone else's and every bit of emotion is expressed through a single glance? She again said to me, picking up my hand, "How are you?" and I started to cry. I told her that I didn't know what had gone wrong to cause me to be on the other side of the side rail but that being on this side was very scary and I didn't like it and wasn't prepared for it (as if we are ever prepared for a diagnosis of cancer). She sat holding my hand and was quiet, nodding that she was hearing every word I was saying and just letting me vent. I rambled on and on about how I worried about the status of my lymph nodes, that I had a 12-year-old child to raise, that I thought I had been a good nurse and empathetic to my patients but that this experience was more profound and life altering than I could express in words. Tears streamed down my face like a faucet that could not be turned off. Myckie cried too at this point. Never saying a word, just holding my hand and listening.

It was now 11:05 p.m. The unit clerk came to my door and sternly said, "Myckie, you are late for giving report." Myckie never turned around to even acknowledge her presence in my room. She never took her eyes off mine. She replied, "Tell them to wait. I'm taking care of a patient." I will never forget Myckie. She could have simply come in, changed my IV bag, emptied my drains, and left that night. She could have seen I was emotional and gotten me a sleeping pill as "the cure." But she didn't. She gave me what I needed most and what she had the least of to give—she gave me her time. I've written and had several articles published about Myckie. I expect any nurse who takes care of cancer patients to be just like Myckie. If they aren't, then I want them to get another job out of the nursing profession.

I didn't sleep all night.

I didn't want to miss a moment of my life.

I didn't sleep all night. Feeling very much in touch with my mortality, I didn't want to miss a moment of my life. My doctor had told me he would come by at 6:15 a.m. to do a dressing change before going off to surgery. My husband was to come in at 9:00 a.m. to take me home. My door opened at 6:00 a.m. though and through the door walked my husband. I was surprised to see him and reminded him that he was 3 hours too early and I wasn't able to go home yet. He said he couldn't sleep without me in the bed and decided to come in early to be with me. Before I could think through that he didn't have a special security pass for coming in that early, the door opened again and through it walked my surgeon. My surgeon did not look at all surprised my husband was there. He said, "Isn't it great that Al is here bright and early to help me do your first dressing change?" I was stunned and numb. Unable to speak. Frozen sitting on the side of the bed. The surgeon had my husband kneel down in front of me so his face was only about 10 inches away from my chest. My surgeon had me sit on the side of the bed and he sat beside me. As he peeled off the dressings from my chest I could feel the coolness of the air on my chest, and I thought to myself that I've never felt this naked in all my life. I was very scared. Frightened about what expression on my husband's face I might see. He looked up at me and gave me a big smile and said, "Baby you look fine. We are fine. You look just fine. You are my transformed woman." I still couldn't speak though. If I could have, I would have shouted "TAKE OUT YOUR TEETH!" I've still never seen that man without his teeth. As you might have guessed by now, after I left the doctor's office my husband and surgeon spoke and decided that my waiting 2 months for Al to see me was too long. They decided as a team to jump start the situation for me. I was mad at them both for about half an hour and then realized they had done the right thing for this patient.

I went home with two drains I called my booby traps. I had been a woman with "bodacious tah tahs" but now only had one "tah." My mom stayed with us for several days to help me. She looked worried constantly and totally overwhelmed by this experience. She and Al would put me in the shower (because I insisted upon washing my hair each morning) and shroud me inside a hefty bag with a hole cut out for my head to poke through. I looked like a Halloween costume that had gone wrong in some way. It was still startling to look down and see my toes on my left foot. Something I hadn't been able to do since age 13.

I returned to the hospital to get the drains out and have the pathology report reviewed with me. Clear margins. Six nodes removed, all cancer free. Hormone receptor negative. I also sent my slides to Vanderbilt to double check that all was well. Though wonderful to hear good news, I didn't want to take it at face value.

CHAPTER FOUR

My New Life with Betty Boob, Then Bobbie Sue

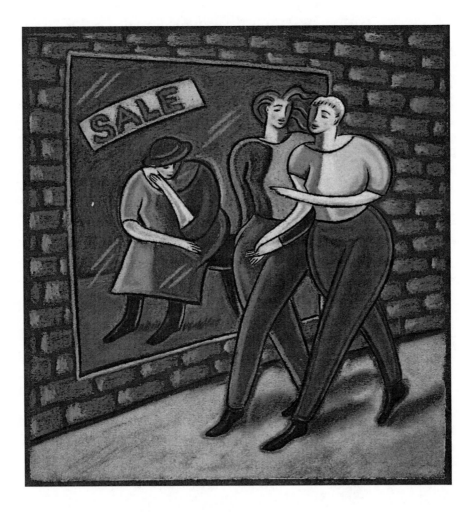

Six weeks after my mastectomy surgery, I was ready to be fitted for my breast prosthesis. I took my mom with me for the fitting. She had fretted so much about everything that had happened. I hoped that her seeing me with my silhouette whole again would relieve her mind. I told her, "You know mom, getting a breast prosthesis is like getting a puppy. She is going to be my bosom buddy. I'm going to take her everywhere I go. So help me think of a name for her." We tested out several names en route to the mastectomy supply shop and settled for the name "Betty Boob." Mastectomy supply shops are given subtle names to let you know what is on the other side of the door. Names like, "We Fit," "Perfectly You," "Just Like Me," "Breast Friends," "Nearly You." It is important to find a shop that has a certified fitter. There is an art and skill to getting the proper-fitting prosthesis and mastectomy bra. So call ahead and ask if you are in need of such a service. There are many sizes, shapes, and even variations on the skin tone shades to select as your new breast. Having a professional to help with this, however, is key. Getting properly fitted for a mastectomy bra is equally as important. When done well, there is no way someone seeing you pass by them, or even hug them for that matter, would be able to tell you have a Memorex version of a breast resting on your chest.

I wore Betty Boob right out of the store like a little girl wearing new red shoes. I decided to send out adoption notices that I had gotten Betty. It included her size, date of her birthday, and such, and one of my girl-friends mailed her a gift. It was a ceramic Christmas ornament shaped like a baby bottle inscribed with "Betty Boob's 1st Christmas, 1992." We keep it displayed in the living room year round and consider it a good substitute for my breast being in the pickle jar.

I felt whole again and walked tall once more, all 5'2" of me. It was virtually impossible for someone to tell that I was wearing an externally worn breast prosthesis. Betty slept in the bathroom at night in her box and was strapped on every morning inside my mastectomy bra. Before long, Al was lightly touching around my incision when we were intimate, and he managed to create a phantom limb type sensation that was comfortable for me and felt similar to touching my breast that was gone. We decided it wasn't necessary to avoid touching that side, so he did.

I did develop phantom limb sensation. Some women do but few talk about it, perhaps fearing they are losing their mind. Just as people who have lost an arm or leg may tell you that they still feel like their limb is there and believe they can actually wiggle their fingers or toes that are missing, I had the same sensation for my breast. No, I couldn't wiggle it or anything. But it felt like it was still there. Periodically my nipple would feel like it was being pinched or feel itchy. The pinched sensation I could deal with, but the itchiness was another issue. Where do you scratch to get relief for an itch that technically doesn't physically exist? This required repeated exploration. After a year I discovered that the nerve for my nipple was in my armpit. If I scratched there when my phantom nipple itched, it would usually relieve it.

The 1st annual Komen Foundation's Race for the Cure in Baltimore was held a few months after my surgery.

It was exciting and emotionally overwhelming at times to be among so many women with pink hats and t-shirts saying they too were survivors.

A year after my first mastectomy, I discovered a lump in my right breast that was different from the cyst that had formed before. I had surgery to remove it and, though benign, it contained atypical cells. Enough tissue was removed that Betty Boob was now a size too big to match with my natural breast, so she was downsized. My surgeon said to me "I predict that you will be back again. Your breasts are trying to tell you something." Not the words you want to hear by any means. Sure enough, he was right. Less than a year later, at age 40, I had another bad mammogram and underwent a second mastectomy. We informed friends and family members about the news by telling them that "Betty Boob was getting a roommate and we wanted help in choosing a name for her." It also became an effective way to neutralize the discussion about cancer treatment. People felt more comfortable asking me "how are Betty and Bobbie Sue" rather than asking how I was dealing with this cancer thing again.

Three weeks after my second mastectomy, we took Laura over to spend the day at Al's mom's home. They were scheduled to bake cookies for the church. Al and I decided to spend the day together and drive up to Pennsylvania to look at the scenery and enjoy one another's company. We drove for about 3 hours when I reminded him that we needed to turn around to head back, because Laura would be finishing up soon. He never even looked at me while driving. He said, "We aren't going back. At least not right now. I made us reservations in the Pocono Mountains where the honeymooners go. We are up here for the weekend." I was stunned. "Where is my suitcase?" He informed me that he didn't pack one for either one of us. Just had my toothbrush in his coat pocket and that was it. He didn't plan on us leaving the room. He said, "I've read before if you lose one of your senses, like your sense of sight or sense of smell, your other senses become more intensified. Maybe the same thing happens to your erotic zones. It is my mission to prove this hypothesis in the next 48 hours." (And he did!) It didn't mean that my breasts weren't important to us anymore. It was the realization that our sex life wasn't dependent on them or any body part for that matter. The closeness that we felt that weekend was extraordinary. I think that it perhaps was because we were both so very aware of how precious life it and that it can be taken away from us without warning or our permission. We had survived together another cancer experience and were celebrating my survivorship.

I now had options with my breast size, having now done a second mastectomy. I could technically be whatever size I wanted to be. So I got several sets of prostheses to wear—one set matching up with my original size and another set that was smaller—40Cs. My cancer cells were hormone receptor positive the second time, so hormonal therapy became part of the treatment plan, which it had not been before. Wow. Hot flashes, night sweats, and vaginal dryness were no fun, but I focused on the purpose, to be cancer free. I was buying Astroglide at Rite Aid regularly, and I suspect the pharmacist thought I was holding orgies at my house. I'd joke with Al and tell him to not walk so fast because if I attempted to walk too swiftly I feared my inner thighs would catch on fire. The clinical trial I

I've read before if you lose one of your senses, like your sense of sight or sense of smell, your other senses become more intensified. Maybe the same thing happens to your erotic zones.

was on also caused some hair loss, which added to my frustration, but again I kept focusing on the mission with my family's encouragement. I didn't want to have to revisit this disease a third time. Today my treatment would have been different, a sign of improvements that have happened over the last decade. I can understand and empathize with women taking hormonal therapy and feeling their quality of life is not at all what it should be. Efforts are underway to reduce these unpleasant side effects going forward, which will be welcome to thousands.

CHAPTER FIVE

Breast Prostheses—Their Many Functions and Purposes

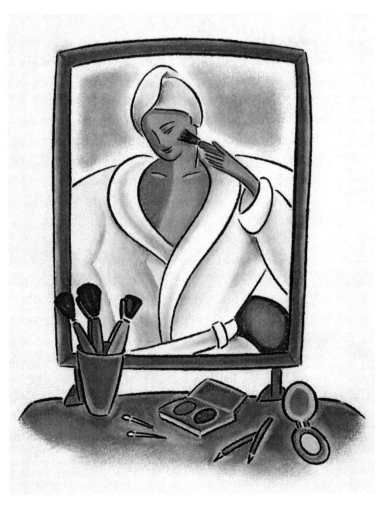

A breast prosthesis is defined as an externally worn breast form designed to serve as a replacement for a breast taken away as an outcome of mastectomy surgery. Breast prostheses have additional meaning though. They serve to replace a valuable part of a woman's body, and though not functional in the way we think of a prosthetic arm or leg for helping someone physically with activities of daily living, they are designed to make us feel whole again and does a pretty good job of it.

I have a great deal of respect for the manufacturers of breast prostheses. I had the opportunity to tour a factory where they are made and was impressed with the care and precision that goes into their design and final creation. I even mentioned to the company that it would be worth their while to stick a little piece of paper in the box with the prosthesis that said, "Finishing touches by Lisa," just so women knew the effort exerted in making each one perfect. I became an advisor and "test driver" for this company, providing input on designs and wearing new models.

Women have told me about the "additional uses" for their prosthesis and mastectomy bras:

- You can stash money in the mastectomy bra pocket for safe traveling.
- You can also stash drugs in them for traveling (I didn't ask what kind).
- A 3-year-old boy used his mother's prosthesis as a hill for his GI Joe doll to rest on.
- Dogs confuse them for chew toys.
- Cats think they are something to exercise their paws (and claws) on.

- They serve as a protective cushion in the event you are stabbed in the chest.

An 8-year-old accompanying her curious sister, age 5, at a health fair came over to my breast cancer display table. As the younger one looked at a prosthesis lying on the display table and inquired what it was, the 8-year-old quickly said, "Don't you know? That's a large nose with a wart on it."

A few years ago I was asked to give a presentation to some important people coming to Hopkins to hear about the program I had created in the Breast Center called "Waking Up Transformed"—how to improve the surgical experience for women undergoing breast cancer. We had created a series of changes regarding the care and treatment of women with this disease so that they felt in control on their day of surgery, had low anxiety, knew everything that was going to be happening to them and with them, and would have little discomfort post-op and be nausea free. This would basically be a male audience. It was the only time I've ever thought I was going to be nervous while giving a presentation.

I wanted to do a good job representing the Breast Center, which was fairly new at the time, in my director's position. I spoke to a girlfriend in Florida before the big day and told her of my anxiety. She said, "You will do great. As a matter of fact, I'm going to mail you something to wear that day that will give you such confidence that you will give your best presentation ever." So I told my husband that I suspected she would send me earrings or perhaps a scarf. But no—when the box arrived from Florida, in it was stick-on nipples for breast prostheses. An unusual gift to say the least! But they came with no instructions and no adhesive. I showed them to my husband and he recommended using Elmer's glue on them. No! I may not want to wear them all the time. He looked at them again and said, "Just put a few drops of water on the back of them. I think they will suction right onto the prostheses without any adhesive." I tried it. It looked like it worked, but I didn't take them for a "test drive" before wearing them for my important speech. I also went out and bought a sheer navy blue silk shell to wear that day. After all, there was no sense in me wearing stick-on nipples if no one could see them, right? I figured the gentlemen would say, "Wow. I thought both her breasts were gone but I think I can see her nipples." And, of course, I would be picturing them sitting there in their boxer shorts.

Well, the big day came and I got myself dressed and really thought I looked pretty hot, like something out of a "Sex in the City" show. You could just barely see the protrusion of the nipples through my silk shell. My speech went great! I did use my arms a lot pointing at my slides. At the end of my presentation I expected the chairman of the committee to thank me and dismiss me but instead he said, "Lillie, we are so pleased to see the work you are doing in the Breast Center here. What a perfect role for you. Come sit beside me for the rest of our meeting." Golly! Was I having a good day, or what? I had on stick-on nipples, my speech went great, and I was honored with being asked to stay for the rest of their meeting. Life was good! Because I was feeling a little flushed, I then made my next mistake and took off my jacket as I sat down, now just sitting in my sleeveless silk shell and skirt. Coming around the table on a lovely china plate were cookies. As the chairman passed me the plate, I reached over to my right to take it. When I got the plate square in front of me, I looked down and on my dessert plate was one of my nipples. I was in shock, the plate now shaking in my hands. The chairman looked at my dessert plate and said, "Oh, I didn't see that they had those thin wafer cookies. That's my favorite cookie. Do they have any more?" I continued to stare at my plate and said, "Gee, it's my favorite too and I think I'll save it for later." I then picked up the nipple and put it in my skirt pocket. He looked at me quite confused. I now said, "Sir, I'm going to go to the restroom. I'll be right back." I stood up and was walking around bent over looking like Groucho Marx, as I retraced my steps looking for what I feared would be my other nipple. I found nothing so I went down the hall to the restrooms. I got myself undressed and discovered that it was my left nipple that had migrated over to the pocket of my mastectomy bra. This pocket is underneath my arm. So as I reached for that doggone plate of cookies, the nipple fell out. The right nipple was right at the edge of the right mastectomy bra pocket. Good grief. I nearly had two nipples on that plate. I returned to my seat, both nipples now securely in my purse, and was quiet for the rest of the meeting.

When I got home, I yelled at my husband. "You don't know a thing about stick-on nipples! You know absolutely nothing!" Then I told him what had happened. He said, "Well babe, I'm glad that you are a quick thinker." I said, "What do you mean?" He said, "Well, let's face it. If you hadn't thought quickly that man might still be chewing." Yikes! Wouldn't that have been embarrassing? I can see me doing the

Heimlich maneuver on that man now. Surely material for the front page of the *Baltimore Sun* newspapers!

I never wore the nipples again. They live in my lingerie drawer. Each morning I say "Good morning girls. Goodbye girls." When I told my girlfriend what had happened, she said she had forgotten to send the temporary adhesive that went with them and would mail it now. I told her to save on postage and not bother. I would be nippleless and happy for it!

Another interesting experience was wearing a bra called a permaform. It's a mastectomy bra with the prostheses built right into the cups. It's also great for wearing in the summer when humidity is high. Silicone prostheses can be quite hot, and this prevents those issues. You throw the whole thing in the washing machine. Quite clever. On a hot day when I was taking our daughter to tour University of Maryland College campus and learn about their program offerings there, I decided to wear this bra. Under normal circumstances that would have been fine, but a storm blew in, causing a terrible downpour of rain that just wouldn't stop. I was sure that due to this weather they would show us a video of the campus in a nice dry room. I was wrong. The woman who came out to take us on the 2-hour walking tour, which we had waited on a list 4 months to get to do, was dressed like she was about to do a commercial for the cover of a salt box: yellow raincoat, yellow hat, and yellow umbrella. She said, "Is everyone ready for the tour?" There was no alternative videotape.

There were 32 of us scheduled for this tour, but 26 people walked out, saying they had no plans of getting soaked to the skin to walk the campus grounds. Because my daughter badly wanted to stay, I agreed to do the walk despite the weather. I did have two umbrellas but no other rain gear with us. That was a mistake. By the time we had reached the fourth building, not only could I pour water out of my shoes but my "breasts" had taken on water as well. The built-in prostheses are made of some type of foam. The weight of the water was causing my breasts to shake themselves down my chest as I ran from building to building. Once inside, I would try to hoist the breasts back up. This of course didn't look very ladylike. Laura was mortified. The tour took 3 hours instead of 2. Waterlogged, tired, and having an unusual form of water weight gain, when the tour came to a close and we got back to our car, I stood outside of the vehicle and literally rang out my breasts, water pouring onto the ground at my feet. Laura said, "Mom, I will never be able to go here. They will remember you from today." So another lesson learned: Don't get caught wearing a permaform bra in the rain or you will be sorry. I must have looked like I had the droopiest breasts ever. I don't know what people thought when they saw me ringing them out. Oh well. No one would have believed whatever they went home and said either!

I also was the "test driver" for some companies that manufacture breast prostheses. One that I tested for them contained liquid silicone. The prostheses were lighter in weight and fit the contour of my chest wall nicely due to the liquid silicone conforming well. The manufacturer hadn't anticipated what would happen to the prosthesis on an airplane or in a city of high elevation like Denver, Colorado. So inadvertently, I let them know what could happen. They bubble, and the air bubbles cause swelling, taking you up more than an additional cup size. Interesting experience and sensation. You can literally become perkier and bigger in a matter of about 10 minutes. I had to knead the breasts to help get the air bubbles out and pray that they wouldn't explode like Lena's air version had. As a result of this "test drive," some changes were made in the manufacturing process to prevent air from getting into the hoses while the silicone liquid is placed in the prosthetic shell. Live and learn.

Another interesting experience with Betty Boob and Bobbie Sue happened in Chicago. I was there to give a speech. The speech was being audiotaped, and it was decided to place a portable microphone on me rather than use a stationary mike. The portable one, however, had a very heavy battery pack, much heavier than I was accustomed to using. It actually weighed 3 pounds. I was wearing a dress that day rather than a skirt, which would have provided me a waistband for anchoring the battery pack. So they decided to unzip the back of my dress part of the way and attach the battery pack to my bra, where it fastened in the back. Why I allowed them to do this remains a mystery to this day. I wasn't using my head. Nor were they. Of course they didn't know that I was wearing my faithful permaform bra that evening either. Very lightweight. Too lightweight for attaching anything heavy to it. So as my 2-hour speech progressed and I walked around the stage, my breasts started moving, upward, on my chest. The weight of the battery pack pulling on the bra strap from the back was causing the breasts to lift up in the front. Every few minutes I would wiggle around and try to pull them down. I have no idea what the audience thought was going on with me that evening. A woman's breasts riding up around her chin is not very attractive. But if left unattended, I surely would have looked like I had a huge goiter in my throat.

Wearing swimmer's prostheses can also be a challenge for some. They were for me. I had gotten swimmer's prostheses to wear before they were really perfected to become swimmer's prostheses. The first set was made of foam and took on water, pulling my mastectomy bathing suit down, literally exposing part of my incisions. So I concluded that this set was for show and not for water sports. The next set I got was made of Styrofoam, again not conducive for wearing in water. I couldn't have drowned if I had wanted to. They functioned like a pair of buoys. My third set that came along a few years later worked better. Not ideal but at least something that would allow for swimming. I had chosen different names for my swimmer's prostheses—Esther and Esther's sister (named after Esther Williams).

CHAPTER SIX

Supporting Others Having Breast Reconstruction

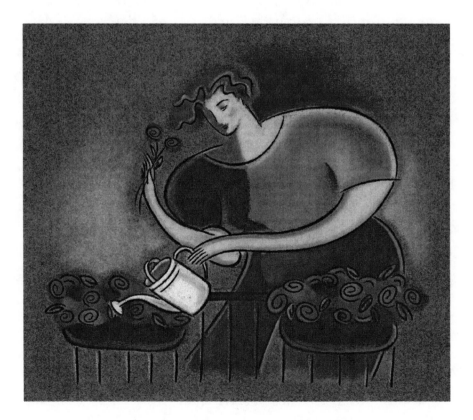

I was not the type to discourage others from having breast reconstruction because I wasn't able to do so. On the contrary, I was the patient advocate and encouraged women to look at all of their options. A girlfriend in California was considering doing reconstruction after having had mastectomy surgery 3 years prior. She e-mailed me and called me, wanting to know my opinion about it. I encouraged her to pursue it if this was what she wanted to do. There was no reason not to go for it. She was worried that I would think differently of her because she felt she needed to do this for herself to feel "complete." I told her that I was part of her cheering squad now to root her on to do this. She was relieved. The week of her surgery I mailed her a present and addressed the box to "Marilyn's new breast" with her address. Contained inside was a t-shirt. Over the right upper chest area it said, "I was the winner of the national wet t-shirt contest." Over the left upper chest it said, "So was I." What a perfect gift to welcome her new breast into this world. She called me and told me that she wore it to work her first day back. What I never told anyone was that I had purchased two of these shirts and kept the other one for myself, buried on the bottom of my lingerie drawer. I never wore it, but it was there in case the day came that I felt "qualified" to put it on.

Quite a few other friends who I had gotten to know well and who were breast cancer survivors also began embarking more on reconstruction, and again I rooted them on just as I had Marilyn. I felt happy for them and frankly a little sad for me, but I always focused on the act that I was thankful to be alive and to have weathered this disease more than once. That was enough for me.

CHAPTER SEVEN

The Right to Choose Reconstruction

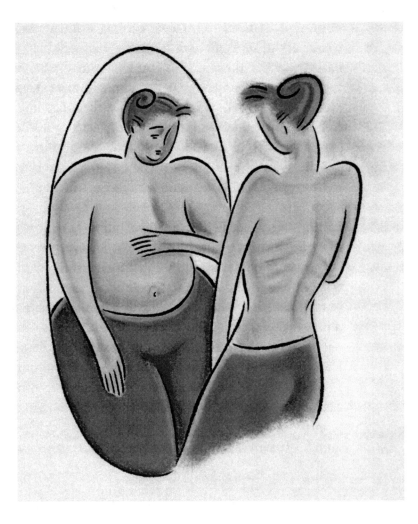

My work in the Johns Hopkins Breast Center as the administrative director was very rewarding. This was the career path I chose shortly after my second round with this disease. I went home satisfied every day and still do, knowing that I've helped someone who has just become a club member with me. Usually, we don't know why bad things happen to us and make a list of them with the anticipation that perhaps we will ask God when we join Him what the learning lessons were from each of them. I was blessed in feeling no need to add this experience to that list. It redirected my nursing career path in line with taking care of other women who ended up wearing the same type of bra I did. I take care of women from all walks of life and all stages of the disease. I counsel patients about their surgical options and discuss with them the pros and cons to assist them with their decision making. This is, of course, if they are fortunate enough to be in a situation to make choices. Most women today can make such health decisions. This also means that I see the surgical outcomes of women after lumpectomy, mastectomy, and mastectomy with reconstruction.

In 1998, after much effort, a federal bill was finally passed to ensure insurance coverage of breast reconstruction as a consequence of breast cancer. I provided testimony to get this bill passed and felt really good about that. My testimonial was a bit unusual or certainly not mainstream. For 3 previous years this bill had been denied. It was voted a big "no" with the rationale that this was cosmetic surgery. I was asked to go to Capitol Hill and provide testimony as to why I felt it was a woman's right to have reconstruction after losing her breast(s) to cancer, so I wanted to prepare myself by reading through previous years' testimony. I believed there was no sense in repeating what had been said before that didn't work. The testimonies were all basically the same—women talking about the importance of their self-image and psychological well-being provided to them with reconstruction. Obviously, this hadn't cut any ice with legislators in the past. So before venturing to Washington, DC, I contacted 16 insurance companies to find out if they covered testicular implants for men who have had testicular cancer. All 16 did. I decided to use this as my testimony, saying, "Gentlemen, it is now our turn." The bill was passed.

In 1998, I held a special fundraiser with proceeds from the event going to cover expenses for Dr. Maurice Nahabedian (fondly known by his patients as Dr. Mo). The purpose of his trip to Europe was to learn a new breast reconstruction method called DIEP flap, for deep inferior epigastric perforator flap. This procedure takes tummy tissue and fat but leaves all the muscles preserved. This is accomplished by stripping out of the muscle tiny perforators and reconnecting those blood vessels up in the chest area. This procedure, therefore, is a true transplant. The tummy tissue and fat are molded into a breast and serve as an amazing Memorex version of a woman's breast. This technique requires learning how to do microvascular surgery. I was thrilled that our patients had a new state-of-the-art option available to them. This new surgery lifted restrictions we previously needed to recommend to women having the traditional TRAM flap procedure (TRAM flap uses the abdominal muscles to reconstruct a breast). As years went by, the surgical outcomes of skin-sparing mastectomy with the DIEP flap reconstruction became even more impressive to me. Many women reported nerve regeneration. Although different from breast sensation, they did have some feeling restored to their new breasts. Fascinating.

Each year I saw my various oncology doctors. For the first few years I mentioned that I still wanted reconstruction one day. Then, at some point in time, I stopped asking, expecting the doctor(s) to bring it up to me. No one did. "How are you doing?" they'd ask. "Fine," I'd say. "Any problems?" they'd reply. "No, not really," I'd tell them.

We brought on board a new medical director, Dr. Ted Tsangaris, in the Breast Center in March 2002. He was a surgical oncologist who specialized in breast cancer. Having a reputation as a skillful surgeon, he was academically talented and was a wonderful leader and team player. Patients adored him, and this was well known. I saw newly diagnosed patients with him just as I had with our previous medical director. I quickly began learning his routine. For women needing mastectomy surgery, he encouraged consultations with our plastic surgery team to discuss reconstruction options. At first, I worried he was being too forceful about discussing reconstruction options. I soon realized he did have the patient's best interests in mind. He told me when we discussed this privately that "when a woman is diagnosed with breast cancer, all she can focus on is survival. 'Let me live. I don't care if I have breasts or not.' She probably does care, though. She is born with two breasts and has the right to have two breasts if medically it is safe for her to do so and it doesn't impact her treatment and outcome. Therefore, she should see the plastic surgeon and talk about reconstruction options."

At that moment, I realized that I had yearned to have breasts again but was doing as most of our patients do— I was waiting for my doctors to bring it up to me. The last time I had brought it up to my doctor was in 1998 when I mentioned that Dr. Mo was traveling to Europe to learn how to do DIEP flap reconstruction. The response was, "That sounds interesting. Good for him." What I wanted to hear was, "Is this something you want to possibly pursue for yourself?" I didn't hear those words, though. And frankly, why should I? I am one of the most assertive women you'll ever meet. I am down-right aggressive when it comes to making sure that our patients' needs and desires are addressed and heard. So, no doubt, my doctors expected me to take the initiative and speak up. But I didn't because I was functioning as a patient and there was, ironically enough, no Lillie Shockney to be my patient advocate and have my desires heard and taken seriously. How ironic.

Wanting DIEP flap reconstruction didn't mean that I had overcome my anesthesia problems that had prevented me from pursuing anything in 1992. My anesthesia problem had continued to be something I had to work around. (Implants didn't interest me either.) I wasn't an ideal candidate for reconstruction anyway, having had multiple abdominal surgeries as well, making the traditional TRAM flap a bit tricky. I had had five previous abdominal surgeries before my diagnosis of breast cancer. Three out of five times I had respiratory arrests immediately after the operation, either in the recovery room or out on the nursing units. No one liked putting me to sleep, and no nurse wanted the responsibility to take care of me during this phase of recovery.

My father has had similar problems, though not quite as severe. In April 2002, he needed a total knee replacement, and I spent a great deal of time with anesthesiology to try to decipher what would be safe to give him so his surgery would go well. He had a 6-hour procedure and sailed through it, spending the night in the intensive care unit for precautionary reasons only. This opened the door to discussing with anesthesiology my personal history and what options they might be now able to offer me. A friend on the anesthesia team carefully reviewed my records and determined that sodium pentothal and Phenergan given in combination might be the culprits to cause my respiratory system to crash. Propofol would be a good alternative, with a 15-second half-life, and an overnight stay in the intensive care unit for observation. Now, suddenly, choice had been restored to me. I didn't have the choice in 1992 or 1994 to do reconstruction with my mastectomy surgeries. I only had desire. I met with Mo Nahabedian and told him I wanted to be evaluated for DIEP flap reconstruction. After examining me and talking with me about my personal situation, he felt I was an excellent candidate.

My brain went into overdrive now. Was it okay for me to pursue this? Did I deserve this opportunity? Was it too late? I always tell my patients it is never too late and that they have the right to be anatomically whole; a woman has the right to choose what is best for her. It is necessary for her to not focus on anything but herself and what she really wants. But I was struggling with giving myself permission to pursue it. Who would take care of patients while I would be on medical leave? This haunted me. I rarely took off blocks of time because of this chronic problem: feeling guilty if I let a patient down while I was away, no matter what the reason.

When I told my husband what I was considering, he became very concerned. "It sounds risky. I don't want anything to happen to you. I've nearly lost you before. Aren't we okay? I think we have a great sex life. Don't you? Am I doing something wrong?" I assured him that we were fine. Now I was being offered options—to choose or not to choose reconstruction. I wanted to do it. When I pressed him about this, he agreed that he, too, missed my breasts. I prayed about this for many days. What should I do? Is it okay to pursue this? Am I being selfish?

I was leaving church one evening and asked God to please give me a sign that it was okay to proceed with the reconstruction surgery. As I arrived at my car and turned on the ignition, playing on the car radio was the song "Sexual Healing." The first full verse I heard was, "You're my medicine, come on and let me in. I can't wait for you to operate." It was the sign I needed, rational or not! I drove home and announced to my husband that I was going to get on the operating schedule for 6 months from then to do the reconstruction surgery over the Christmas holidays. This would give me 6 months to plan out my work schedule and hopefully recruit help from our survivor volunteer team to pinch-hit for me. Yes, I'm a planner. I wanted to decipher a plan that would have me away from patients the shortest period of time and help ensure that those who were diagnosed and treated while I was out would have someone there with them filling my role. I kept my plans a secret from everyone but my husband. A month later I told our daughter, then 22. She worried about the surgery, telling me, "Mom, you look fine as you are." I had a heart-to-heart with her, explaining that just as she enjoys her cleavage now, I

I asked God to please give me a sign that it was okay.

missed having my own. I waited until September to tell my parents, who were quite stunned by the news. Dad asked, "Are you doing one or two?" I told him, "Dad, I might do one big one right in the middle— Ms. Uni-boob." He was overwhelmed with everything and simply said supportively, "Okay."

As the weeks approached to my surgery date, December 5, 2002, I felt like I was preparing for the birth of a baby. So I began to refer to my future new breasts as "the girls." "The girls are being delivered December 5th. We will bring them home from the hospital on December 9th." I started looking at bra ads in the newspaper again. I hadn't done that for years—10 years to be exact.

I started looking at bra ads in the newspaper again.

I went public with my decision to do delayed reconstruction at the beginning of November, announcing it at our Survivor Retreat and received applause and support for my decision. And just as Mo predicted, breast cancer survivors who had had mastectomies without reconstruction in the past began calling, requesting evaluations for "the same surgery Lillie is having." I was clearly clueless until then of the impact my own previous breast cancer surgery had had on other women and their decision to have or not have reconstruction.

CHAPTER EIGHT

My Final Steps Through Transformation

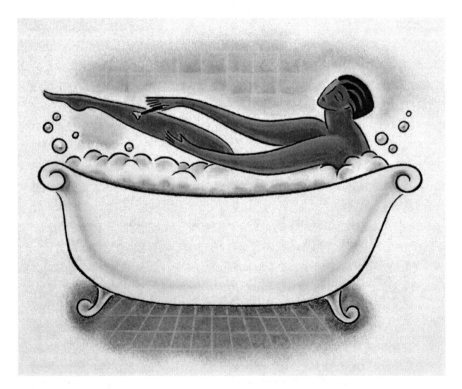

As I showered on the morning of my surgery, I rubbed the bar of soap across my chest for the last time. I had always said that when I looked down in the shower, I didn't see that my breasts were gone. I saw that the cancer was gone. I realized that soon I would be seeing two healthy surgically created breasts that would be cancer free and remain that way for life, hopefully. Wow. I also realized that every person taking care of me, from checking me in at the registration desk to putting me to sleep, operating on me, and caring for me post-op all knew me, worked with me, and several were my closest friends. What an extraordinary journey I was taking with them. I had asked Ted Tsangaris to be with me while I was put to sleep, feeling this would be my most nervous period. He agreed to do so but exceeded my expectations as a dear friend by serving as Mo's first assistant in the operating room, helping throughout my surgery from beginning to end.

The surgery lasted more than 12 hours. Laurel Moore, also a dear friend, was my anesthesiologist who, ironically, was with me for my first mastectomy. She was in the preop room at the time of my first mastectomy when I had removed my bra and said, "I'll never be able to wear this again." Now she was with me again, as I removed my mastectomy bra to put on my hospital gown and heard me say, "I won't have to wear this bra again. I can't believe it." I requested to listen to the song "Sexual Healing" as I went under anesthesia. Though certainly not a religious song, it had spiritual meaning for me.

Once asleep, I knew that my hospital gown would be lifted up to my neck, exposing nearly every inch of my body. I had prepared typed signs to wear, which were taped to my chest and abdomen—some comic relief for the OR staff. Over my right mastectomy incision it said, "Please super size me." Over my left mastectomy incision it said, "I'm here for a front end realignment." And over my navel it said, "Dear Santa, thanks for bringing me cleavage for Christmas." Undoubtedly the signage brought a laugh to the OR team. I hoped it would reduce their stress a bit as they began working on one of their own Hopkins' family members. I also realized that this would be for me yet another form of transformation surgery.

"I'm here for a front end realignment."

With the exception of initial laryngeal edema that was quickly under control in the ICU and sciatica that had flared up from being on the OR table longer than anticipated, I did well and awakened in the ICU with family at my side. Mo and Ted spent the night at the hospital to be doubly sure I did fine and to be sure that the circulation to my new breasts continued. (Wouldn't you know it—a woman's fantasy is to have two men to sleep with whose focus is on her breasts and I looked like crap and felt like hell. Oh well.)

A Doppler was used hourly to listen to the blood supply in each of my new breasts. It reminded me of listening to a baby's heartbeat in utero. Wawoosh. Wawoosh. My mother heard a different sound though—wow, wow, wow. She said, "That's the sound I hear them saying because they are so happy to be here!" I went home on day 4 with six drains that would stay in for a week. My tummy was flat and tight and, initially, if I tried to stand up too suddenly, I felt like my vagina was bungee jumping off my chin. This feeling subsided as a few more days passed.

The day my drains came out and I was able to get in the shower without tubes and devices in my way, I took a bar of soap and slowly washed my new breasts with tears streaming down my face. It was a profound moment. The girls and I were home and doing fine (and they were each capable of holding a bar of soap under their mammary fold).

During my recovery I received lots of get well cards and flowers from friends, who were excited that I had at long last done something for myself. They were not the traditional get well cards that one normally receives following a big surgery though. The majority were related to giving birth! "Congratulations on the birth of your twins!" The flowers arrived in pink baskets, ceramic baby carriages, and balloons celebrating the birth of my baby girls! Hysterical! When one of the florist's delivery men arrived twice in the same afternoon delivering flowers to me, he said on his second trip, "Gee, for having newborns in the house, your house is really quiet." I was so tempted to "show him the new girls" but somehow resisted.

Anxious to be back with patients, I returned to work early, at 4 weeks post-op. Al and I resumed sex at 5 weeks. (Yes, a little ahead of doctor's recommendation of 6 weeks.) We quickly turned into a pair of honeymooners, test driving my new body often. He told his brother, "I feel like I'm sleeping with another woman and have my wife's permission."

I requested Al to take a torso shot of me every Saturday morning when I got out of the shower, beginning at 1 week post-op. This may sound like a strange request, but I wanted to actually be able to see the changes the new breasts went through from week to week. They begin looking rather flat and firm and actually more laterally positioned on the chest. Over a period of weeks they plump up and medially shift inward. Amazing. (This may one day be a line dance. Everyone up for the Medial Shift!). My mistake, however, was assuming my husband knew what a torso was. I did ask him, "Do you know what a torso is?" He said, "Of course." I now realize I should have said, "What is it?" I didn't. So every Saturday morning he took my photo.

When I was 10 weeks post-op, I took the roll of film to Rite Aid for 1 hour developing. Yes, another mistake. When I returned an hour later, there was my film still being processed, coming out of the developing shoot for everyone to see. A tall man around age 35 was standing at the counter looking at the images as they scooted down the shoot, in clear view. He looked intrigued. When I saw what he saw, I was horrified. The images were of me from my neck to my knees. He said, "Look! Those are pictures of a naked woman up there!" I said to him calmly, "Don't be silly. You are in Rite Aid." The young clerk put the film in the envelope without really even looking at them and gave them to me. I paid for them and went home and yelled at my husband for not knowing what a torso was! You could, however, see what I had hoped—the changes the breasts make rather quickly over time. Of course, the photos also showed things not intended to be seen too.

I named my new breasts Jessica and Sleeper. Yes, this requires an explanation as to how these names were selected. My left one is Jessica, named after Jessica Rabbit in the movie, "Who Framed Roger Rabbit." The right one is named Sleeper because Dr. Tsangaris told me there was difficulty getting the vessels to connect on that side. "She was a sleeper, but finally woke up" after much effort and the vessel connection was complete. In my dreams I would imagine that they both could communicate, Jessica being very brazen and flirty and Sleeper being very shy. One day I hope to have them formally speak to the public like the crash dummies who get us to wear our seatbelts. Perhaps Jessica and Sleeper could inspire other women to get mammograms, do breast self-exams, and see their doctor annually for clinical breast exams. I wrote an article for Yahoo.com called "If My Bra Could Talk." We need to find as many creative ways as possible for women to reduce their fear of this disease and do the right thing when it comes to monitoring their breast health.

I wrote an article for Yahoo.com called "If My Bra Could Talk." We need to find as many creative ways as possible for women to reduce their fear of this disease and do the right thing when it comes to monitoring their breast health.

Our daughter took me bra shopping—an event that should have been videotaped. Three hours of laughter and twice a few tears. She went through the department store bra sections like Grant through Richmond and proceeded to show me what a bra can do for a woman's breasts today: lift them up, push them together, pull them apart, add a cup size, deepen cleavage—you name it and there is a bra that could do it. And the color choices were amazing. My last experience with bras before mastectomy bras was wearing a Cross Your Heart minimizer bra I had ordered from a catalog. Now I'd be wearing bras that had names, color, and designer configurations that really should come with an operator's manual. Not to mention the role reversal of my daughter, now 23, fitting her mother for a bra. (I also privately ordered a few items from Frederick's of Hollywood, too.)

In April 2003 I had my nipple reconstruction done. Al had written on the calendar "Nipples coming!" I didn't realize how important this procedure was to him until that day came. My pager went off at 10 a.m. for a phone number I didn't recognize. Assuming it was an error in paging, I called the number thinking I would let them know they had punched in the wrong pager. The person answering the phone said "emergency room." Now I was totally confident that paging me was an error. I said that I thought that someone had entered in my pager number by mistake when the voice on the other line said, "Is this Mrs. Shockney?" My heart raced now as I confirmed it was. "Your husband is down here with chest pain. Can you come down here please? Oh, we hear you are getting new nipples today, is that correct?" Good grief.... "We think he is just experiencing angina. A little overly excited about getting your nipples I guess. Come down so the cardiologist can talk to you about him." I rushed downstairs. There was the cardiologist with him. He came over to me and said, "I think he is fine. We want to keep him overnight though to be safe. So you are getting nipples today, right?" Well heck, why not just announce it over the hospital intercom system? I asked if it would be better for me to cancel the surgery and concentrate on him. The doctor said, "Absolutely not. If you cancel, he will think he is sicker than he is. Get the nipples done and return to him with new nipples." So I did.

It was a 22-minute operation with a local anesthetic. I actually had it done between morning and afternoon clinic. For this procedure, my husband had gotten me pink-sequined pasties to wear to mark where I wanted my nipples to go. I returned to him afterward. He now was situated in the coronary care unit, oxygen in place and cardiac monitors on. And what did he ask when I arrived? You guessed it—let me see them. And so I did, which resulted in his monitor going off and the emergency team coming into his room before I could get my clothes back on. One of the residents said, "What is going on in here?" Before I could answer, a nurse I didn't even know said, "Oh, she got her nipples reconstructed today." I don't even want to think how any of this was documented in his medical record. He was discharged the following day.

To prevent prematurely flattening the nipple, it is recommended to not wear a bra for a while. This resulted in me looking like the "erotic oncology nurse." So I bought callus cushions at the drugstore that look like small flat donuts, perfect for sticking over the nipple to protect them. By stacking them and sticking them on, two deep, they were level with the tip of the new nipple and fit fine inside a soft cup bra. Great! (Of course without my bra on, my breasts looked like they were going scuba diving, having their goggles already on.)

In October 2003, I had my areola tattooed. The doctors were amazed with how much lidocaine I needed to numb my new breasts. I have nearly full sensation in my right breast and about 60 to 70% in my left breast. Wonderful. I'm officially finished with my transformation and am thrilled with the results. Though it has been more than 3 years now, I still surprise myself when I look in the mirror. I still smile with joy in the shower every morning when the girls and I get wet and soapy. And perhaps I am even more pleased than most women would be because I have mourned the loss of my breasts, was resolved I would never have them again, and was given the gift of choice at long last—to choose or not to choose reconstruction. Was it worth the wait? You betcha. In my case, waiting gave me the

opportunity to experience a newer method of reconstruction superior to the traditional flap reconstruction
still done throughout most of the country. This newer
method along with free flaps has become the standard
for Hopkins' patients and is a wonderful improvement
that has been made over the last decade.

CHAPTER NINE

A New Home for Betty Boob and Bobbie Sue

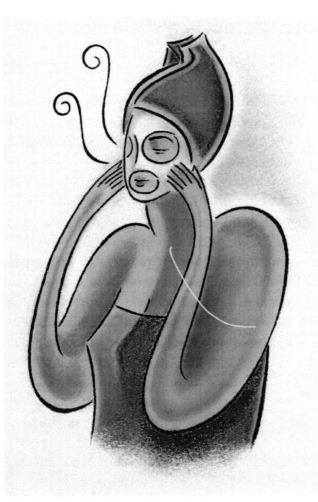

What did I do with Betty Boob and Bobbie Sue, my breast prostheses? I wanted to select someone very special to receive them. I took my time in selecting a patient who would be having bilateral mastectomies without reconstruction. The patient I selected didn't undergo reconstruction because she had no time for recovery, having five young children she was raising, none of which was even her own. (They were born with a variety of medical complications since their mothers were heroin addicts.) She had outpatient surgery mastectomies so that she could get back to the children as soon as possible. She was large busted like myself. She came to the clinic post-op, hunched over wearing a large sweatshirt with her cotton batting breast forms underneath. She was clearly lacking self-confidence in her appearance. I presented her with my breast prostheses and mastectomy bras and properly fit her to ensure they would work for her. She literally wore them out of the Breast Center like a child wearing new shoes from the shoe store. She stood tall and confident again and said, "I think I might be able to catch a man with these." She hugged me tight for giving her this special gift of an important piece of me from an important time in my life—my bosom buddies. I realized at that moment as we were embracing that my new breasts were actually hugging my old prosthetic breasts. It was as if my old girls were perhaps saying, "Welcome to Lillie's. We know you will enjoy your stay. We did. She is full of life and love and energy like no one else we know. You will meet many newly diagnosed women with breast cancer just as we have over the last decade. She will utilize you as she did us, giving women hope and reminding them that this is a disease that is emotionally charged and tests our psyches. We'll come by to visit periodically with our new owner. Again, welcome."

CHAPTER TEN

Counseling Patients about Breast Reconstruction

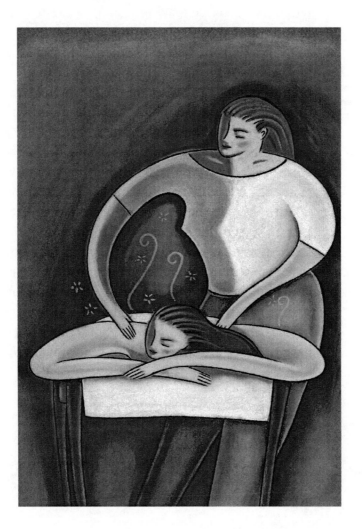

Having now had a lumpectomy, two mastectomies, and delayed reconstruction, I am able to discuss with patients personally as well as professionally all their options. Some women worry that having reconstruction will cause them to develop recurrence of the disease, but this is not the case. They also worry that it may mask a new cancer growing. Also not true. They do, however, need to take their time in deciding what they want to do. Sometimes women ask which method has the quickest recovery time. This isn't the way to choose reconstruction options though. They need to remember they are making a short-term investment of healing and recovery time for a long-term gain. So faster may not be better for them. How they want to look a year from now is how to answer that question. So my counseling focuses on this, including what their lifestyle habits are, hobbies, activities, and what their relationship has been with their breasts. That may sound silly, but how a woman views her breasts and what role they have played in her life speaks volumes to me. If she tells me they are her best feature versus telling me that she has never been happy with them, that is a significant piece of information to know. Remember that women have the right to choose. It is a personal choice whether or not to do breast reconstruction. It can be done usually at the time of (skin-sparing) mastectomy surgery, but it also can be done later if necessary or desired. Sometimes we simply have to be reminded that choice is a woman's right.

They need to remember they are making a short-term investment of healing and recovery time for a long-term gain.

Some "flapper advice" from an experienced flap patient to a prospective one!

1. Remember you are a work in progress. The reconstructed breast will start off feeling firmer, lying

flatter, and perhaps more laterally positioned than you anticipated. Give her time ... she will plump up, soften up, and medially shift in all by herself in the coming weeks. (When I explained to my husband that my breasts would medially shift together, he thought I was describing a new line dance—Everyone up for the Medial Shift!)

2. Gentle massage of the flap starting at 6 weeks post-op can help to regenerate the nerves. You are welcome to recruit "help" for this exercise.

3. Initially, you will feel very full and very tight in your tummy. Actually, during your hospital stay you will void a lot, getting rid of excess fluid that was given to you intravenously during the surgery. Over a period of several weeks, your waistline will reappear and your tummy will soften and get even flatter. Amazing.

4. Don't spend money on expensive bras too soon. A camisole with a shelf bra in it is the best alternative for the first 6 to 8 weeks. Wait until your new breast(s) has really settled in before getting fitted for new bras. If you did unilateral flap surgery (just one side), more than likely your old favorite bras will fit just fine too. Of course, an excuse to get new bras should never be turned down.

5. Nipple reconstruction also should not be done in haste. Wait at least 3 months post-op so the breast is settled. You don't want your new headlights not lining up, for heaven sakes.

6. Tattooing usually happens 1 to 2 months after the nipple reconstruction is done. Commonly, the shade chosen will be a little darker than the desired finished color. This is due to there being some fading after the procedure is done.

7. Sometimes to create the symmetry desired, some tweaking is needed afterward. This can consist of liposuctioning to even out the two breasts or some nips and tucks around the tummy tuck area. Not everyone needs this though. I didn't need any touch-ups after my surgery.

I had the opportunity to meet with a patient and her husband before her having mastectomy with DIEP flap reconstruction done. She was from another country originally, so English was not her first language. They asked to meet with me to review several things, including having some "personal questions" (to quote her husband) about the recovery process. I knew that meant he had questions about sex. His wife was recording everything I was saying. I told her it wasn't necessary to do this because this information was written down in the preoperative teaching documents she and her husband had been given. He told me, however, that she processed the information better by writing it down. Fine. He asked good questions—"When can I squeeze her new flap breast?" When she is 5 weeks post-op, you can begin gentle massage. "When can we resume sex?" You can resume intercourse at 6 weeks but I recommend having her on top at first to avoid pressing on her tummy incision. She hadn't spoken a word. She looked over at him. Said nothing. He said, "She's never done that before." I told her it was time she tried it! She wrote down, "Massage breast—5 weeks. Intercourse—6 weeks but me on top. It looked so funny seeing this information being recorded. As we got to the end of our time together and stood up, I hugged her and said, "Actually, I think you will feel well enough to resume oral sex at 3 weeks post-op if you want to." She looked at her husband and said, "Do you want me to write that down?" He said, "Heck, yes!" She did. She wrote "oral sex—3 weeks." As they were exiting my door, he instructed her to go to the elevator and wait for him there. She did as instructed. He came back over to me, gave me a bear hug, and said, "I'm so glad we came in to see you today and so glad you are open about discussing sex with your patients. We've been married 18 years and have never had oral sex. She wrote it down so now I know it's going to happen!" He burst out of my room on that note. Holy schmoley. That will teach me to phrase my recommendations differently in the future!

CHAPTER ELEVEN

What Does the Future Hold?

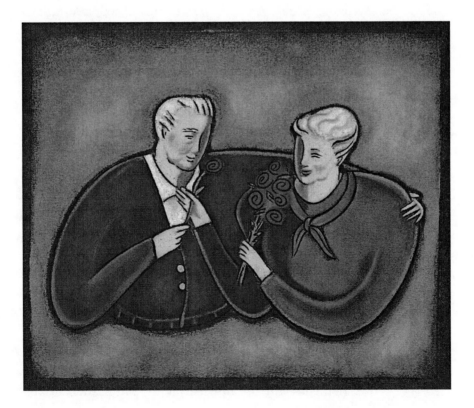

Data available from Tumor Registries nationally confirmed that in 2002 there were 5.6 million women who were survivors of breast cancer, alive and thriving. In 2005 there were 250,000 women diagnosed. It is projected as baby boomers come into midlife that this number will climb to be potentially as high as 500,000 in the year 2012. That's a lot of women and a lot of breasts. If we look worldwide, there were 1 million women diagnosed in the year 2000, and it is estimated it will be 2 million women in the year 2030. So don't ever consider yourself alone in this battle. Eighty-five percent of the women diagnosed in the United States today will be long-term survivors like me. The mortality rate has been slower, going down over the last few years as well—another sign that we are diagnosing the disease sooner and have created better ways of treating it.

500,000 women diagnosed in the year 2012.

The future looks hopeful too for future generations. Targeted therapies are being developed: designer drugs, laser ablation, and even vaccines. The day will come that this disease will be listed in medical books next to polio, a cured disease. I will always encourage people to hold tight to their faith and to their sense of humor as they take on whatever lies ahead of them, related to breast cancer or any other life-threatening illnesses. I have a plaque on my wall at home that says "Laughter is God's hand on the shoulder of a troubled world." It's true. Staying "abreast" of the latest developments in research related to breast cancer will also provide us all additional peace of mind and hope for the future ... for your grandchildren's future.

The future looks hopeful too for future generations.

I consider it a privilege to get to take care of other women who will end up wearing my bra in their future.

This is one of the most vulnerable times in a woman's life, and being able to make her journey the least physically and emotionally traumatic that I can is my mission. It's one of the reasons I believe I was spared twice and allowed to survive this disease—to fulfill that mission.

I am also privileged to work in the finest institution in the country and with some of the most amazing dedicated and talented doctors and nurses who specialize in this disease. We have a team of remarkable plastic surgeons who specialize in DIEP flap, all artists in their own right; surgical oncologists dedicated to breast cancer surgery, striving to conserve a woman's breast whenever medically possible and as is her desire; medical oncologists; radiation oncologists; radiologists; genetics specialists; and pathologists, all specializing in this disease and providing compassionate care. I could be in no finer place to receive care or to provide it. In 2006 I was given a faculty appointment in the Department of Surgery, which was a great honor for me. It will enable me to get more involved in clinical research as well, with a focus on improving quality of life for women during and after breast cancer treatment.

One initiative I am working on to improve the quality of care for women undergoing breast cancer, diagnosis, and treatment is the development of national quality standards for breast cancer. There remains wide variance across the country related to how a woman is diagnosed and treated. It's hard enough to cope without the extra burden of having to ensure you are in good hands. This should not be an issue, but it is for many. Breast cancer diagnosis and treatment may not be available at every institution in the future. You wouldn't go to just any health care facility if you needed a heart transplant, right? You would seek out a center of excellence that has demonstrated a track record for being very successful at doing heart transplants. Well, one day I hope the same may apply for breast cancer. Watch for more news on that initiative in the future.

I do a great deal of traveling across the country and even internationally to help raise awareness about this disease and promote improvements in quality of care. You may find me on a college campus assisting with a Breastival™ or at a Bra Run with Leather & Lace, a female motorcycle club. I'm frequently spotted at American Cancer Society events, Komen Foundation seminars, Y-ME conferences, Young Survival Coalition meetings, Breast Centers across the country, and Living Beyond Breast Cancer events locally, regionally, and nationally. I hope to see you there! I also personally participate in many walks, including the Avon Walk held in Washington, DC, each year. I'm easy to spot. I'll be wearing my pink scrubs and shaking pink pompoms as our team of Johns Hopkins walkers crosses the finish line each day. So come join me. And I'll be at these events and talking to groups large and small, wherever needed until we no longer need to do races and walks and talks...until there is prevention and a cure.

My daughter was interviewed a couple of years ago regarding breast cancer. One of the questions she was asked resulted in me crying when I heard her confident answer so boldly stated and without hesitation. The reporter said, "Are you frightened at the possibility of one day perhaps also getting breast cancer?" She responded, "No, I'm not. I actually expect to get it. But my mother has shown me how to beat it. Actually, she showed me twice to make sure I got the message." Wow...profound words for me to hear. And it's true that her risk is higher than the average population. I have had two primary breast cancers and her grandmother, Al's mom, died of inflammatory breast cancer. To complicate matters further, Al was recently diagnosed with malignant melanoma, also a type of cancer known for being potentially genetically linked to breast cancer. My parents are also cancer survivors— prostate and uterine. So hormonal-driven cancers surround her. She is well informed though and always at my side for every breast cancer event I do. She remains our greatest joy in life. I believe we have done a good job in rearing her. But I would give my life without hesitation to spare her going through breast cancer herself. As a mother I can endure anything happening to me, but not to my child, no matter what her age.

My mother obviously feels the same way. She was a basket case through my first diagnosis and treatment. I think she wanted to shove me back into her womb, assuming I hadn't cooked long enough the first time. She had no control over what was happening and couldn't fix it or do it herself for me. Very frustrating and emotionally exhausting. The second time around I anticipated her being worse, but instead she was the rock I've always known her to be in a crisis. We discussed this at length afterward—that her being steadfast and calm speeded up my recovery. She explained that the first time she didn't know what to expect, what to do, and felt totally lost and out of control. The second time she had experience under her belt, understood the disease and its treatment, and knew how to constructively help me rather than be a burden on me.

She wanted to help other mothers going through the same turmoil and asked me to help her find a support organization for mothers where she could periodically volunteer. I searched and found nothing. The Internet was new in 1994. There were only six cancer websites, four with bulletin boards where messages could be posted. I posted a message on each one saying, "I'm seeking a support group for mothers who have daughters with breast cancer. If you know of one, would you e-mail me back privately?" Twenty-four hours later there were 116 e-mails in my inbox each basically saying the same thing—"I saw her post. Don't know of a group, but if you find one would you e-mail me back for my mom?" I called my mother and said, "Ma! I have found an organization that provides support to mothers who have daughters with breast cancer." She said, "Great, where is it?" I told her, "There isn't one so we are going to create one. It's you." Six weeks later with the support of Senator Barbara Mikulski, we founded Mothers Supporting Daughters with Breast Cancer, which is now a national nonprofit organization helping mothers (and daughters) nationally and internationally. (As Hannibal said, "If we can't find a way we will create one.")

CHAPTER TWELVE

Experiences That Reinforce I Was "Chosen" to Work in the Breast Cancer Field

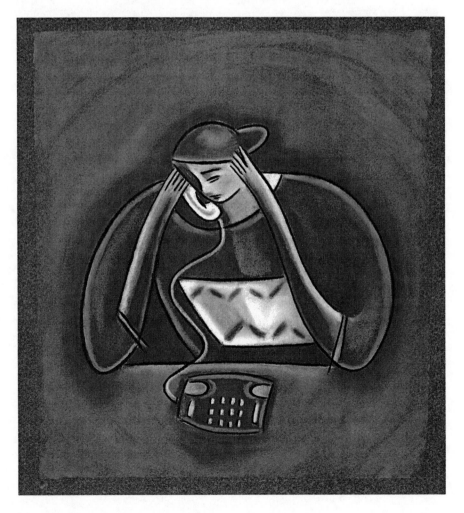

I know that many people get up in the morning and as they are going to work or just arriving there they say to themselves, "What am I doing here. I don't want to be here. What am I supposed to be doing with my life? I don't think this is it." I'm blessed to not be one of those people... though there was a time that I believe I was. It was long ago, so long ago I don't even remember the details anymore. What changed that situation? Being diagnosed with breast cancer. Though breast cancer wasn't on my list of goals I intended to achieve while on this earth, having been dealt the cancer cards, I decided to do as I had been taught by my parents, especially my mother: take the bad and find the good in it. That can take some time and some need for reflection, but we are all capable of finding the pearls if we choose to look. And I did look, and oh what a wealth of pearls there were for me to uncover and cherish.

Being diagnosed with breast cancer and being given the opportunity to survive provides each of us with the chance to step back and assess how we are spending our time and begin to look more closely as to whether what we are doing is really contributing to this world in a positive way.

Being diagnosed with breast cancer and being given the opportunity to survive provides each of us with the chance to step back and assess how we are spending our time and begin to look more closely as to whether what we are doing is really contributing to this world in a positive way. We are in touch with our mortality ahead of schedule and begin to realize that life is more precious than we recognized or conceived and needs to be valued and not taken for granted. Relationships take on a different tone, some perhaps ending and others becoming more meaningful.

I knew when I was still recovering from my first mastectomy surgery that I was destined to devote my personal and professional time exclusively to this disease and the women who end up wearing my bra in the future. A physician friend called and asked if I would be willing to talk to one of his employees who had just been diagnosed. As soon as I got on the phone with her and started offering her medical information and support, I knew that this was where I was meant to be. In the Breast Center at Hopkins, I help patients and their families cope with the shock of the diagnosis, make decisions about their treatment, empower them with information, and see that this is a disease that can be overcome.

This chapter provides you a look into my workday and private life in a candid way as I share patient experiences with you. Frankly, a book could be devoted to just this alone. In some cases it was hard to select which stories to share. I think as you read through them, however, you will find what I have found, the joy in helping others. These simple acts of kindness are those that anyone could do if they chose to and sought similar opportunities to be in a position to help others. I go home every night knowing that I've made a difference in the lives of people I've encountered through my day. In some cases they are people I never actually met. I spoke to them on the phone or had e-mail contact with them. They are out there though, and they give me a gift of appreciating my efforts at a time they felt lost and perhaps even without a sense of hope.

The Story of Jo

I was sitting at my desk responding to e-mails one afternoon when my phone rang. I picked up the receiver and provided my usual introduction: "This is Lillie Shockney.

May I help you?" The voice on the other end of the phone was desperate and tearful. "Who is there?" I replied again, "This is Lillie Shockney." "Where am I calling?" I replied, "You've reached the Breast Center." "But where? Which breast center?" I was surprised to think that she was so stressed she wasn't even sure what institution she was calling. I simply responded, "The Johns Hopkins Breast Center." She then said, "Can you help me?" I said yes, without even asking yet what her problem was and then asked her to describe her situation to me. She tearfully explained that she was a new mother, age 34, and her baby was just a week old. She had been diagnosed with inflammatory breast cancer that had spread to her bones and lungs. She had told her OB doctor numerous times during her pregnancy that her one breast was red, hot, and hard. He had placed her on antibiotics, which she had taken for more than 3 months without relief and steadily watched her breast get worse. She had complained that her hips hurt and her ribs hurt. Still she was ignored and told that all these symptoms were related to her pregnancy.

When she delivered, by C-section, she complained more about her ribs hurting than her new abdominal incision. Still her doctor didn't listen, but the anesthesiologist did. He was concerned and requested a chest x-ray 24 hours after the baby arrived. There were pathological fractures to her ribs. She had metastatic disease, and it was everywhere. She was told that there was no treatment. It was too late and to go home and spend time with her new baby. They estimated she would live about 3 to 4 weeks at the most. That conversation had taken place just days before her call to me. So she said, "Please tell me Hopkins can do something. I don't want to die and leave my baby. I don't want to leave my husband alone to raise her. Please help me to live, even if just for a year."

I instructed her to come to Hopkins the next morning, and when I hung up with her I wondered what I could do to buy her time. Was it possible? What would it take? Was it unrealistic to give her a sense of hope? I worried during the rest of the evening and night. I arranged for her to see a surgical oncologist as well as a medical oncologist the next morning. She arrived with her husband in the clinic. Her baby was being taken care of by her mother at home. She walked toward me and I put my arms out to embrace her, being as careful as I could to not squeeze her too tight as to avoid hurting her brittle bones more. She walked like she was 98 years old. Her husband looked like a deer caught in a car's headlights—scared, bewildered, and very nervous. He was just 28 years old. They had been married 3 years. This was their first child. He acted a bit odd though when he met me. He pointed at my name badge and shouted, "IS THAT YOUR NAME?" I said, "Yes, this is my name on my ID badge." A few minutes into the consultation with the team he turned to me again and said, "Is that YOUR name on the badge?" I again replied that it was. Thirty minutes later he asked me yet again about my ID badge. "I need to know if that is YOUR name on your badge." I replied again, "Yes, this is my name. The badge says Lillian Shockney. That's my legal name. Everyone calls me Lillie. Please call me Lillie too." Jo, the patient turned to him and said, "Honey, I told you last night that I called and got connected to this wonderful nurse and she said that Hopkins could help us so we are here and they are going to help us. Help me. Don't you remember?" He nodded his head yes but still stared at my name badge.

We were able to help Jo. We got her underway with chemotherapy in 48 hours. Though she understood her prognosis was poor, she was appreciative of any time that treatment could afford her. She wanted to be here as long as possible to raise her new baby. We set a goal initially of 6 months. Once we saw that her disease was responding to chemo, the goal was changed to 1 year and then 2 years. I saw Jo and her husband regularly. She even was able to eventually have a mastectomy and took a break from chemo and radiation for 2 months to spend time with her family and enjoy being a mother. It was a huge celebration when her child turned 2—a point in time that frankly none of us thought was initially achievable.

Her husband called me one evening at my home. Usually, he would call if there was a problem, but this time he was calling for a very different reason. He wanted to thank me for helping his wife and him and making it possible for his wife to live as long as she had. He realized that she probably wouldn't make it to their little girl's next birthday, but he appreciated the time they had had together and wanted to tell me a story. He asked if I remembered the first time I had met him. I told him that I remembered him accompanying Jo to the breast center and that he was very stressed. He said, "Yes, and I kept asking you about your name badge." I had actually forgotten that part until he mentioned it to me again. I replied, "You were very nervous that day. I didn't think much about it." He said, "Well, I've thought a lot about it and want to tell you a story and hope you won't think that I'm out of my mind. My grandmother lived with me when I was growing up. She and I were very close. She was wheelchair bound since I was a toddler but never let life get her down.

She was a remarkable and loving woman. Even after Jo and I married, I still stopped at my parents' house every day on my way home from work to see her. That's how close we were to one another. She became very ill toward the end of Jo's pregnancy, and we knew that she was going to die. I was with her that evening at her bedside, a moment I will never forget. You see that was before we knew that Jo had cancer, before all of the bad news came. It was 2 weeks before the baby was born. Grandmom said to me, 'I wish I could live long enough to see your baby come into this world. This new life that will soon be here. But I can't and I accept that as God's decision. But I hope to return to you as a guardian angel over all three of you and you won't necessarily know me by my face but you will instead know me by my name.'" He paused a moment and then said, "Her name was Lillian. You see, my wife wasn't calling Johns Hopkins the day she got connected to you on the phone. She was calling her mother in need of a good cry, and instead of reaching her mother who lives in a totally different area code than yours and has a totally different phone number, I believe my grandmother fulfilled her promise to me and connected Jo to you." I shivered as I heard him describe this to me. No wonder this young man was so focused on my name badge when he met me. He had never shared his grandmother's dying words with Jo either. The additional irony is that I was named for my grandmother.

Jo lived another year, passing away shortly after their daughter's third birthday. She accomplished her goals. She wanted to survive long enough that her child would remember her. To this day her little girl tells her daddy that every morning early before sunup she sees her mommy's face, just her face, and hears her voice say, "Good morning sunshine!" So that tells me that Jo is serving as a guardian angel over her little girl now. That gives me a sense of comfort and peace too.

If ever I had a doubt that I was in the right profession and doing what God wanted me to be doing, all doubts left my mind that night. And though the story sounds far-fetched, it is all true, and I feel blessed for having been the chosen one to help this family.

The Story of Claudia

I've been known to offer people help in unusual ways, which is something else I get from my mother. I've heard my mother say that she will help a total stranger cross the street even if they don't necessarily want to go. Well, I am cut from the same block of wood. We have international patients come to us for breast cancer treatment. This is not unusual at all actually. One patient who had corresponded with me via e-mail initially was Claudia. I helped arrange for her to come over from Germany. She was scheduled for a mastectomy with a tissue expander. Her husband was not able to be with her at the time of her surgery, and the thought of someone doing this without support was more than I could bear. Though it is not unusual for me to see a patient off for surgery and be one of the first faces she sees in the recovery room, I broke the rules and offered to drive the patient to the hotel and stay with her overnight and help take care of her. After all, this is not a time to be alone. I also wanted to help her manage her drains. She was most appreciative of my offer.

We were set for her big day when I got the flu. Usually, I still go to work when I'm sick, but I was more ill than I had been in a long time. My family doctor grounded me to home, as was certainly the right medical decision to make for me, but I was distressed I was going to be letting down this patient who was counting on me to be with her. So I called my mother at 11 p.m. and said, "Mom, I need your help. There is a woman here from Germany having mastectomy with reconstruction tomorrow morning at 7:30 a.m. I was scheduled to be with her before her surgery and see her in recovery afterwards as well as drive her to the hotel and spend the night with her. Can you substitute for me and do this?" Now under normal circumstances someone else's mother may have asked a bunch of questions and challenged me as to why I was extending myself to patients in this way, but not my mother. What was her reply? She said, "What is her name and what time do you want me to come over in the morning?" I told her to arrive by 6:00 a.m. This meant that she would be getting 3 hours sleep since she lives 2 hours away from the hospital. No problem. She was going to be my pinch hitter.

So Claudia was surprised and greeted by a woman who was in her mid-70s and looked like an older version of me. Mom gave her hugs and kisses as she was rolled off to surgery, the surgeon came out to tell mom how the procedure went as if she was blood relative, the nurses gave mom a quick refresher course in drain management (something she was familiar with having helped me three times with drains), and mom drove her to the hotel and spent the night with her, checking on her throughout the night to ensure all was fine. They bonded as if they were blood. My mother even offered to stay with her a second night, but Claudia was actually doing extremely well on her own and kissed mom goodbye and remains in touch with her to this day. I can't imagine how strange the story must sound to people when Claudia tells the story back home in Germany. She came to Hopkins and a nurse's mother spent the night with her? Go figure.

The Story of Jana

Some patients are amazing in how they take on this disease and accept each bump in the road in stride. Jana was one of those patients. Raising three young children, the oldest being 5, and having a husband who traveled a lot didn't keep her from rolling up her sleeves and taking on her surgery, chemo, and radiation like it was just another hectic day in her life. She was amazing.

Toward the end of her chemo, her counts dropped down very low. Dangerously low. Her temperature spiked, and she ended up in an inpatient bed with us. This was the first time I saw her depressed and anxious and feeling and looking defeated. Her children were too young to visit, and she was too sick to go home. She was also in isolation so there were many visiting restrictions. I had a respiratory bug myself, and although I still came to work I was staying away from patients like Jana who were very susceptible to infections and viruses. We spoke on the phone and she was very tearful. I said to her, "Which direction is your hospital room facing? What can you see outside of your window?" She told me that she could see the Broadway street and the garage across the street next to the outpatient center building. Perfect! I told her to watch out her window and in 15 minutes she would see a cheerleader with pink pompoms on the rooftop of the parking garage doing a special cheer just for her to help her body get her counts back up! I put down the phone, went to our storage closet to get my pink pompoms (doesn't everyone have pink pompoms stored somewhere?), grabbed one of the other nurses in the Breast Center who also is a breast cancer survivor, and said, "Come on, we are heading to the rooftop to cheer Jana up!" It was 18 degrees—not exactly cheering weather. But it didn't matter. I was on a mission!

We ran back and forth across the rooftop yelling and saying cheers—J-A-N-A-Her counts WILL go Up today!! A man parked his SUV up there while we were doing our cheers. As I looked across the street and on the fifth floor of the Weinberg building where I knew Jana was located, I saw a patient pressing herself up against the window in her room waving back at us. It was Jana. Despite a long distance of space between us, she saw us and we could see her! When we finished the cheer and proceeded to get back into the elevator to go downstairs, the gentleman who had parked his vehicle up there near us declined to get into the elevator with us, clearly thinking I was a nut case. Oh well. Jana really appreciated the gesture, and 3 days later she was well enough to venture home again.

The Story of Bill and Mary

I get many e-mails from people in need of help. Some are simply questions about a breast abnormality they are experiencing and need to know what to do and others are heart wrenching, as was the case of an e-mail I received from a man named Bill. He explained that his wife, Mary, age 34, had been battling breast cancer for more than 3 years. It was now in her brain, bones, and liver. She was in the hospital and was sleeping a great deal. He outlined the entire treatment that she had had, listing every surgery, chemo drug, radiation, hormonal therapy, and how the disease progressed. He then wrote that after they found the brain metastasis she began to have seizures and underwent full brain radiation. Her condition worsened, however, and she was hospitalized. He stated that the doctor asked to meet with him, so he had gone in the night before to see him. The oncologist told him that the drugs and therapy weren't working anymore and it was "time to switch to hozpiss." He said the doctor didn't explain any more and promptly left so Bill opted to go to the Internet, where he found me and wanted to know "how effective is the drug hozpiss on brain mets? I found the drug Herceptin but can't find information on the drug hozpiss."

When I read this e-mail, my heart sank. He didn't know that what the doctor was telling him was unrelated to drug therapy and instead was actually hospice care, helping his wife get closure with her life and die with dignity and be as comfortable and prepared as possible for end of life. He was searching online for a drug to make her well again. I couldn't just e-mail this man back and explain this. It required a phone call. I wrote him back, giving him my cell phone number to call me at whatever hour he read my response.

My phone rang at 6:00 a.m. It was Bill, sounding a bit perplexed. He said he was very surprised that "Hopkins would e-mail him a cell phone number to call." I explained to him that his wife's situation was such that it didn't seem appropriate to just send an electronic response and that I preferred to talk with him over the phone about it. I reiterated what he had e-mailed me regarding her treatment and when I reached the point of where he said that the oncologist wanted to meet with him to discuss the future plans, this was where I stopped and asked, "Tell me more about your meeting with the oncologist last night. Exactly what did he say?" Bill again told me the meeting was brief and that he said the treatments she had been given weren't working anymore and it was time to switch to this other drug, hozpiss. At this point, I told him that this wasn't a drug but a program, and it was spelled differently from what he thought. I asked him if he had heard of hospice before and he said he hadn't. I explained that I thought perhaps it was assumed by the doctor that he was familiar and that it probably was so painful for the doctor to have to deliver this unfortunate news that this may be why the meeting with him was so brief. I then explained the purpose of hospice.

Needless to say, Bill was devastated and got very upset. He told me that Mary couldn't die. They had two small boys still to raise and that he couldn't do that without her. I told him that he would need to do it and that he would, for her. And that he now needed to be strong for her so that she could accomplish what she needed to with her boys in the potentially brief time that remained. I then asked him to go to the local card store that morning before returning to the hospital and to explain to the manager his wife's situation. I told him to request that the manager assist him in selecting birthday cards for each boy up through age 21, holiday cards, graduation from high school and college, even cards for their wedding day, and for when their own first child is born. The manager would need to help because many holidays and events such as Christmas are not displayed year round but are kept in their storage room in the back of the store. He then was to go to the hospital and help his wife write one sentence in each of them for each of their boys. What message did she want to tell them as they reached certain milestones of their life? She could still, through these words, be right there instilling her values in them and loving them. They would feel her spirit.

Though Bill cried throughout this conversation, and it was all I could do to not do the same, he said, "I can do this! I will!" He called me the next day and told me that he had fulfilled his assignment, gotten the social worker to help with arranging hospice, and was bringing his wife home from the hospital. He e-mailed me 4 days later that she had passed away and that all the cards were safely placed in a lockbox for the future, and thanked me for my help.

There are times when I just feel too weary to respond to e-mails, and when those moments come I think about Bill and Mary. What would have happened had he not found me and contacted me? What would have happened had I not been candid with him and spoken to him one on one on the phone? No cards, no words of closure perhaps. But that wasn't what happened. Good things resulted.

This isn't the only couple I've given this advice to. I recently received a card from a teenaged girl who just reached her 16th birthday. Her mother had been a patient I had gotten to know well 6 years ago. I assisted that patient myself with writing in these cards for her daughter. The 16-year-old was writing to tell me that she opened the birthday card from her mother and felt so at peace to see her handwriting and read her words of encouragement and love on her 16th birthday. She was writing to thank me, on behalf of herself and her mom. Wow. We never do know when we are creating a memory for ourselves or for someone else.

Other Stories

Singing to patients—So what kind of a song would you sing to a patient having a breast procedure done in the breast center, wide awake, who is feeling anxious? A song from your nursing school says "Do Your Boobs Hang Low?" (Do your boobs hang low? Can you swing them to and fro? Can you tie them in a knot? Can you tie them in a bow?) Yes, that's the jingle I sing to them. It serves as a great distraction from their worries about what is happening to their chest. Whether it is draining an abscess, removing a drain, or something else that results in a few minutes of intensity for the patient, that song gets them smiling and usually laughing. Perhaps one day you, too, will have a chance to sing it to someone.

The joy of telling someone their sentinel node is negative—Although patients are told by their surgeon the results of their sentinel node biopsy, which is done at the time of breast cancer surgery, they seldom remember. The effect of anesthesia and narcotics clouds their memory. So when the patient sees me in the recovery room, this is commonly the first thing they ask me, "What is the status of my sentinel node." What a wonderful thing to be able to tell someone that it was negative. No evidence of cancer found in it. It's like reinforcing in their mind that this disease is beatable. They will live. They can endure. The squeeze from their hand is tremendous. The look of relief on their face is immeasurable. Joy. Thankfulness. The realization that they have gone way up the survival curve, and ridding their body of the source of this disease has been achieved today. They now view themselves for the first time perhaps as a survivor.

The joy of looking at a woman with a reconstructed breast and telling her that she is beautiful—There can be great anxiety for a patient the first time she looks at her reconstructed breast that was done immediately after her mastectomy surgery. The realization that her natural breast is gone and why it is gone can be an overwhelming feeling. The critical eye can expect more than what is realistic when first looking at the new rebuilt breast. Having someone reassure her that she looks wonderful and reminding her that she is a work in progress is an important role I fulfill each day. Her breast is new and needs to settle in and take shape, and it will over time. I tell her to focus on the fact that she is, we believe, cancer free and that she has two healthy breasts now. In some cases the reconstructions are remarkably gorgeous right from the start. Amazing. Some women have even said that their newly built breast looks better than the original version. Always produces a giggle too.

The joy of looking at a woman who has had a mastectomy without reconstruction and telling her she is a transformed woman—transformed from victim into a survivor and radiates having climbed way up the survival curve today as a result of surgery.

The human touch is such a powerful sensation.

The power of a hug—The human touch is such a powerful sensation. It speaks volumes without having to utter a word. Whether it is holding someone who has just learned she has metastatic disease or embracing her when she learns that the sentinel node biopsy was negative, it is powerful moment. I believe that we don't hug enough. Granted I'm an unusual person in that I AM a hugger and do so regularly with patients and family members. I wish more people were comfortable doing the same. I think they are missing out a lot when they don't allow people into their space and share that moment. It's irreplaceable for both people who are intertwined in each other's arms.

Johns Hopkins Breast Cancer Survivor Retreat is an event that happens annually during the first week of November. Helping women re-engage in life emotionally healthier after their treatment is done is the goal of this 2-day overnight stay event. We want to help transform a woman from a breast cancer patient into a breast cancer survivor so she can move forward with her life. Breast cancer is a life-altering experience. There is no doubt about that. But if we support her in the way she needs us to, we can hopefully set her on a path that will enable her to see that her life is more fulfilling and enriching after breast cancer than it was before. This is a weekend filled with emotion—laughter and tears. Even women who swear they "never cry" do cry during these 48 hours together. It is the most exhausting event I do through the year. It also is perhaps the most fulfilling. These women become reborn, and I am given the privilege of being with them at that moment.

Seeing a patient get married—When we see young women coming in who are diagnosed with breast cancer, many dynamics come into play, including how she will ever be able to think about showing a future beau her breast cancer surgery scar, dealing with hair loss and dating, and anxieties about whether she will survive to find love and marry. What a joy to see patients return several years after treatment with a wedding band on their finger and a huge smile on their faces. Sometimes women e-mail me a photograph of them in their wedding gown and will write some message emphasizing that they never thought they would get to experience this day—proof that there is life and love after breast cancer.

Seeing a patient have a new baby—Women are equally distressed if they were hoping to have a family in the future and now have been told their life is in danger due to this disease. Seeing a patient several years after treatment has been completed coming through the lobby toting a bundle in her arms is heartwarming in an indescribable way. There she is carrying the next generation in her arms. A miracle that she didn't believe she would ever get to experience. And yes there are anxieties about whether she may have passed a breast cancer gene onto her child, but the joy outweighs the worries for now. I like to try to reassure patients today that by the time their child really needs to worry about this disease, we hopefully will have it solved.

Avon 2-Day Walk—There are many more stories that I could share with you, but it seems most fitting to end with a story about this event that we participate in annually. Hopkins has a team for the Washington, DC, Avon Walk. Most of these team members are our own breast cancer survivors. They walk 39 miles over 2 days and raise more than $1800 each for their registration fee to participate. It's a grueling yet invigorating weekend in which sisterhoods are formed, and the realization that the monies raised from these events support future breast cancer research, education, and breast care for the underserved makes the event very meaningful. Reading the words written on women's t-shirts is a special part of the two days: "I'm walking for my mom." "I'm walking so my daughter doesn't have to." Wow. This year our team of 21 walkers, most of whom are survivor volunteers in our Breast Center, will be taking turns carrying a pair of pink scrubs that belonged to one of our survivor volunteers, Betsy. Betsy passed away just a few weeks ago. She has always had a presence at the Avon Walks since we began participating in them several years ago. This year, we think of Betsy as our Spirit Walker ... with us in spirit, walking alongside our team, each mile, each step. Betsy will be there. Each team member will have an opportunity to carry Betsy's pink scrubs as she walks, and then pass them along to another Hopkins walker on our team until they cross the finish line...39 miles from their starting point. Betsy will be a guiding force for those who believe they just can't walk another few feet, but with her inspiration I know they can and will.

Thousands of people coming together for the same mission. The same cause. One of our walkers has committed to walk until there literally is a cure. What an amazing commitment to make. My hope is that she won't have to walk much longer.

My hope is that she won't have to walk much longer.

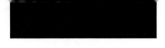

Resources

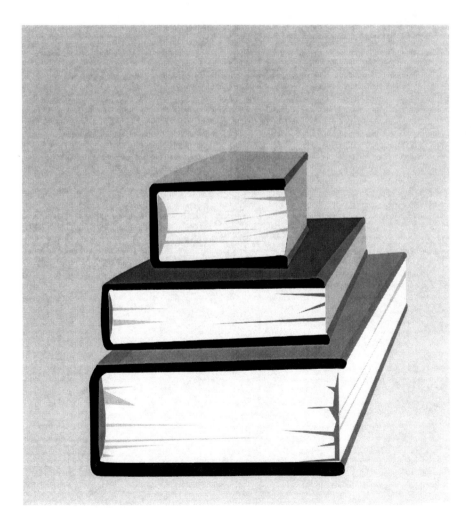

American Society of Plastic Surgeons
*http://www.plasticsurgery.org/public_education/procedures/
BreastReconstruction.cfm*
This organization provides a helpful website that describes the
various types of breast reconstruction and shows anatomic
drawings of how the procedures are performed.

National Cancer Institute
*http://www.cancer.gov/cancerinfo/understanding-breast-
cancer-treatment/page13*
This specific URL of their website offers educational information
for patients and family members seeking information about
breast reconstruction options.

American Cancer Society
*http://www.cancer.org/docroot/CRI/content/CRI_2_6X_
Breast_Reconstruction_After_Mastectomy_5.asp*
1-800-ACS-2345
The URL above is a specific area on the ACS website for reviewing educational information about breast reconstruction.

Cancer Information Service of the National Cancer Institute
800-4-CANCER
http://www.cancer.gov
This organization provides information about all types of cancer, including excellent information about breast cancer, what
it is, how it is treated, and where various treatment options
are provided. You can request free information by calling the
toll-free number.

The Johns Hopkins Avon Foundation Breast Center
410-955-4851
410-614-2853 (Lillie Shockney's Direct Line)
Her e-mail: shockli@jhmi.edu
http://www.hopkinsbreastcenter.org
This Breast Center is one of the few comprehensive cancer centers in the country that offers state-of-the-art breast cancer
diagnosis and treatment. A special feature online is *Artemis*,
Hopkins' electronic breast cancer medical journal, that you can
subscribe to online for free. It is published online monthly and
provides the most up-to-date information about the latest

available research results and information related to diagnosis and treatment of this disease. The website also has sections about diagnosis and treatment information, breast imaging, pathology and breast reconstruction, breast cancer patient bill of rights, and other valuable resource information.

If you plan to be evaluated or treated at Johns Hopkins, you will probably meet Lillie Shockney. She interacts with patients daily and matches the team of breast cancer survivor volunteers with women newly diagnosed based on their age, stage of disease, and anticipated treatment plan. The survivor volunteer, who has already completed the same treatment plan the patient is about to embark on, remains connected with the patient as long as the patient desires, which usually is through and beyond the end of treatment.

Susan G. Komen for the Cure Foundation
National Helpline *1-877 GO KOMEN*
http://ww5.komen.org
This is a national volunteer organization seeking to eradicate breast cancer as a life-threatening disease, working through local chapters and the Race for the Cure, events in more than 110 cities. The foundation is the largest private funder of breast cancer research in the United States. The Komen Alliance is a comprehensive program for the research, education, diagnosis, and treatment of breast disease. You will find information on their website about their mission, the accomplishments they have achieved to date, how you can participate, grants they have funded, calendar of events nationally, and other information. Komen is very big on education about the disease and on ensuring treatment for the underserved.

Mothers Supporting Daughters with Breast Cancer (MSDBC)
410-788-1982
E-mail: msdbc@verizon.net
http://www.mothersdaughters.org
This is a national nonprofit organization dedicated to providing support to mothers who have daughters diagnosed with breast cancer. This organization offers a free "mother's handbook" and "daughter's companion booklet" that provides basic information about breast cancer and its treatment as well as some recommended constructive ways for mothers to provide sup-

port physically, emotionally, financially, and spiritually. The organization also "matches" mothers with mother volunteers across the country based on the daughter's (patient's) clinical picture, age at time of diagnosis, and anticipated treatment plan. The also have a newsletter online and a bulletin board for posting questions. Lillie Shockney is the "daughter" and cofounder of this organization.

Y-Me National Breast Cancer Organization
800-221-2141 (24-hour national hotline)
800-221-2141 (24-hour hotline in Spanish)
http://www.y-me.org

Y-Me is committed to providing information and support to anyone who has been touched by breast cancer. The services listed on this website include a national hotline for women needing emotional support, kid's corner, referral information for approved mammography facilities near you, public education workshops where you will find a listing of upcoming events, teen programs where you can order a video specifically for teenage girls to learn about breast cancer awareness, and a resource library that provides information about treatment modalities.

Young Survival Coalition
155 6th Avenue, 10th Floor, New York, NY 10013
Tel: 212-206-6610
E-mail: info@youngsurvival.org
http://www.youngsurvival.org

The Young Survival Coalition (YSC) is the only international nonprofit network of breast cancer survivors and supporters dedicated to the concerns and issues that are unique to young women and breast cancer. Through action, advocacy, and awareness, the YSC seeks to educate the medical, research, breast cancer, and legislative communities and to persuade them to address breast cancer in women 40 and under. The YSC also serves as a point of contact for young women living with breast cancer.

Breastcancer.org
111 Forrest Avenue 1R, Narberth, PA 19072
http://www.breastcancer.org
Breastcancer.org is a nonprofit organization dedicated to providing the most reliable, complete, and up-to-date information about breast cancer. Their mission is to help women and their loved ones make sense of the complex medical and personal information about breast cancer, so they can make the best decisions for their lives.

Where Can I Get Help with Financial or Legal Concerns?

Accompanying any serious illness are questions and concerns related to expenses incurred as a result of treatment, health insurance questions that can be overwhelming to try to understand or resolve alone, and sometimes even legal questions related to employment or financial matters. Below is a list of national resources to aid you in addressing these types of concerns.

CancerCare, Inc.
212-302-2400
800-813-HOPE
E-mail: info@cancercare.org
http://www.cancercare.org
CancerCare is a national nonprofit organization that provides free professional assistance to people with any type of cancer and to their families. This organization offers education, one-on-one counseling, financial assistance for nonmedical expenses, and referrals to community services.

National Coalition for Cancer Survivorship (NCCS)
301-650-8868
877-NCCS-YES
E-mail: info@canceradvocacy.com
http://www.cansearch.org
This network of independent groups and individuals provides information and resources about cancer support, advocacy, and quality of life issues and helps cancer patients deal with insurance or job discrimination and other related legal matters.

Patient Advocate Foundation
757-873-6668
800-532-5274
E-mail: patient@patientadvocate.org
http://www.patientadvocate.org
This organization provides educational information about managed care/insurance issues and legal counseling on debt interven-
tion, job discrimination issues, and insurance denials of coverage.

About the Author

Lillie D. Shockney, RN, BS, MAS

Administrative Director,
Johns Hopkins Avon Foundation Breast Center
Faculty, Department of Surgery, Johns Hopkins School of Medicine

Ms. Lillie D. Shockney is a registered nurse with a BS degree in Health Care Administration from Saint Joseph's College and a Masters in Administrative Science from the Johns Hopkins University. She has been employed at Johns Hopkins since 1983. Her career has focused on clinical nursing care with a special focus on cancer patients. She also served as the Director of Performance Improvement and Utilization Management from 1987 to 1997. After a personal experience with breast cancer, when she was diagnosed at age 38 in 1992, Ms. Shockney began to contribute additional time to the hospital as a volunteer for the Johns Hopkins Avon Foundation Breast Center. In 1997, she formally joined the Breast Center staff and serves as the Administrative Director, responsible for the quality-of-care programs; patient education programs; survivor volunteer team; community outreach at a local, regional, and national level; webmaster; and patient advocacy. Ms. Shockney is a published author on the subject of breast cancer as well as a nationally recognized public speaker on the subject. She has written four books and many articles on breast cancer. She serves on the medical advisory board of several national breast cancer organizations and is the cofounder and vice president of a national nonprofit organization called Mothers Supporting Daughters with Breast Cancer. She is also the recipient of the Global Business Leadership Award, numerous community service awards, the Outstanding Women of America Award, the Distinguished Graduate for Lifetime Achievement Award in 1997, and in 1998 received the National Silver Medal Award from the National Consumer Health Information Center for her educational material "Breast Cancer—Making the Right Choices for You."

Additional honors include the National Circle of Life Award and the American Cancer Society's Voice of Hope Award (1999), the American Cancer Society's Lane A. Adams Award for Excellence in Caring (2001), the American Cancer Society's Faces of Breast Cancer Award (2002), and the Oncology Nursing Society's Award for Excellence in Breast Cancer Education (2002). In 2003, she was the recipient of the Impact Award from the National Consortium of Breast Centers for her lifetime achievement in making measurable improvements nationally with the treatment of breast cancer. She also was the recipient of the Komen Award from the Maryland Affiliate of the Susan G. Komen Foundation in 2003. In 2004, she was a finalist for the Lance Armstrong Foundation's Spirit of Survivorship Award and also was selected as one of the Top 100 Women in Maryland for her leadership and community service efforts. Ms. Shockney was selected nationally by the Komen Foundation to receive the 2005 Professor of Survivorship Award with the goal of advancing research and awareness on the issues surrounding long-term survivorship of breast cancer. Professor of Survivorship awards are made to individuals who have made significant contributions in the field of breast cancer survivorship. She also has a faculty appointment as an instructor in the Johns Hopkins University School of Medicine, Department of Surgery.

Ms. Shockney is a strong advocate of the value of humor as a beneficial form of complementary medicine and speaks often on this subject locally, regionally, and nationally. Since the summer of 2005, Ms. Shockney has served as an Ask the Expert for Yahoo Health to provide educational content to this website regarding breast cancer. Ms. Shockney also has a personal goal to foster the development and implementation of national quality standards for the diagnosis and treatment of breast cancer here in the United States.

About the Author

CPSIA information can be obtained
at www.ICGtesting.com
Printed in the USA
FSOW01n1158020315
5383FS